LGBTQ-I HOSPICE AND PALLIATIVE CARE

HARRINGTON PARK PRESS

NEW YORK, NY • USA   YORK, NORTH YORKSHIRE • UK

LGBTQ-INCLUSIVE HOSPICE AND PALLIATIVE CARE

A PRACTICAL GUIDE TO TRANSFORMING PROFESSIONAL PRACTICE

KIMBERLY D. ACQUAVIVA

Harrington Park Press
Box 331
9 East 8th Street
New York, NY 10003

http://harringtonparkpress.com

Library of Congress Cataloging-in-Publication Data

Names: Acquaviva, Kimberly D., 1949– author.
Title: LGBTQ-inclusive hospice and palliative care : a practical guide
   to transforming professional practice / by Kimberly D. Acquaviva.
Description: New York, New York : Harrington Park Press, [2017] |
   Includes bibliographical references and index.
Identifiers: LCCN 2016049204 (print) | LCCN 2016050626 (ebook) |
   ISBN 9781939594143 (pbk. : alk. paper) | ISBN 9781939594150
   (hardcover : alk. paper) | ISBN 9781939594167 (ebook)
Subjects: | MESH: Palliative Medicine | Homosexuality | Bisexuality |
   Hospice Care—methods | Health Knowledge, Attitudes, Practice
Classification: LCC R726.8 (print) | LCC R726.8 (ebook) | NLM WB 310 |
   DDC 362.17/5608663—dc23
LC record available at https://lccn.loc.gov/2016049204

Manufactured in the United States of America

For all the lesbian, gay, transgender, gender nonconforming, queer, and/or questioning kids out there. May this book be rendered completely unnecessary in your lifetime by a community of health care providers who can't fathom providing anything other than LGBTQ–inclusive care.

CONTENTS

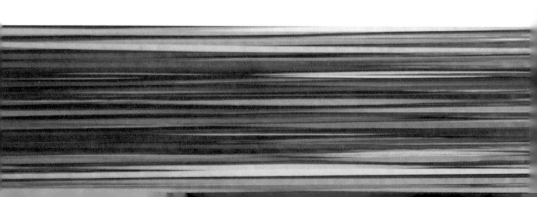

ACKNOWLEDGMENTS

This book would not have been possible without the support and encouragement of my wife, Kathy, and our son, Greyson. Throughout the writing process they cheered me on, made me laugh, and showed me time and again the value of a chosen family one can count on. Kathy's ceaseless enthusiasm for my book project was an act of love for which I will always be grateful. This book is as much hers as mine; without her support I could have never written it. Greyson's relentless positivity, unique ability to find humor in everything, and genuine interest in my daily word counts made every day I was writing this book a joy.

My dad, Phil, shared insights from his experience caring for my mom as she was dying, reminding me that there are so many ways we can make palliative and hospice care better for all the patients and families we serve. The experiences of my mother-in-law, Ann, as a person with Alzheimer's disease, and those of my wife in providing long-distance care coordination for her, motivated and inspired me. My grandmother Eleanore, an emeritus professor, offered valuable support and encouragement throughout the writing process.

Three mentors inspired me and provided much-needed encouragement while I was writing: Dr. Jean Johnson, founding dean of the GW School of Nursing, Dr. Ellen M. Dawson, founding senior associate dean of the GW School of Nursing, and Dr. Stephanie Wright, former senior associate dean of the GW School of Nursing. Jean, Ellen, and Stephanie shaped my career by showing me early on that the key to success in academia isn't grant funding or publications or presentations — it's integrity and servant leadership.

The support of my community at Friends Meeting of Washington also made writing this book a joy. Thanks to the tweens and teens in the Quaker Ukulele Collective, every Sunday was a raucous reminder that there's more to life than work.

While writing this book, I was also fortunate to have a large circle of friends in my Scouting family cheering me on. Each week the Scouts and Scouters of Capitol Hill Scouts Troop 500 inspired me with the way they view the world through the lens of the Scout Oath and Law. Capitol Hill Scouts issued a public, formal diversity statement in 2001, expressing that all Scouts and leaders are welcome, regardless of sexual orientation. It is because of that statement that my son joined Scouting and is now an Eagle Scout. Inclusion truly does make a difference.

My friends from Wood Badge course N6-82-15-1 and N6-82-16-2 showed me over and over again that a future in which all are valued, respected, and included *is* possible. I was writing this book during the six-month staff development process for the course, and the following Wood Badge staffers deserve medals for all the encouragement they provided: Bao-Thuy Nguyen, Shawn Carroll, Christopher Cooper, Dr. Nick Maliszewskyj, Rick Pitterle, Tom DiMisa, Julia Farr, Mike Nepi, John Howlin, Yong Ho Halt, Roger Brow, Bobby Tran, Enrique Gutierrez, Dr. My-Huong Nguyen, Phillip Ramsey, and Stephen Allen. The three youth staff I worked most closely with—Ethan Cooper, Laura Herbig, and Riley Howlin—exemplified the best of Scouting and the best of humanity. The future is in good hands. My fellow troop guides deserve a separate shout-out for their love and support: Scott Bashore, Odessa Benton, Ken Buszta, John Herbig, Ryan Nagle, Thad Palmer, and Mark Serfass. Finally, the members of the N6-82-16-2 Bear Patrol deserve my gratitude as well: Jason Boles, Maria Raffucci Cooper, Bryan Martin Firvida, Dr. Nam Le, Jeff Lepak, and Locksley Moody.

At work, my colleagues at the George Washington University were a steadfast source of support during the writing process. Several colleagues in particular stand out for the extraordinary inspiration they provided: Dr. Steven Lerman, Dr. C. Dianne Martin, Dr. Mary Jean Schumann, Dr. Jessica Greene, and Dr. Ellen T. Kurtzman. I am grateful to Dr. Pamela R. Jeffries, dean of the GW School of Nursing, for granting my request for a sabbatical to write this book.

I could not have published *LGBTQ-Inclusive Hospice and Palliative Care* without the valuable input and feedback of the following content expert reviewers, each of whom read the draft manuscript, provided detailed comments, and validated the content within a month of receiving the draft—a heavy lift they undertook because of their commitment to LGBTQ-inclusive hospice and palliative care: Rev. Vonshelle Beneby, Constance Dahlin, Gary Gardia, Dr. Judi T. Haberkorn, Dr. Noelle Marie C. Javier, Samuel Mullen, and Dr. Martha Rutland. I also owe a debt of gratitude to the hospice and palliative care professionals, patients, and families who submitted their stories for inclusion in the "Provider Perspective," "Patient Perspective," and "Family Perspective" text boxes that appear throughout the book: Dr. Kathryn Almack, Dr. Constance Dahlin, Kunga Nyima Drotos, Gary Gardia, Richard Gollance, Jennifer Hawkins, Rev. Anne G. Huey, Lynne Hunter, Dr. Noelle Marie C. Javier, Jay Kallio, Nick Krayger, Rev. Holly Lux-Sullivan, Vicki Quintana, Steve Shick, and Kathleen Taylor.

Words cannot begin to express my gratitude to Bill Cohen and Steven Rigolosi of Harrington Park Press for their professional advice and assistance in writing, polishing, and publishing this manuscript. Working with Harrington Park Press was truly a pleasure. Bill and Steve invested considerable time and effort in making this book as strong as it could be, and I will always be grateful to them for their support, guidance, and friendship. Many thanks to Patrick Ciano of Ciano Design for designing such a dynamic cover and for overseeing the innovative design and layout of the interior. The cover of this book is proof that designers do their best work when the client's bad design sense isn't an albatross dragging the designer down. Julie Hagen had the onerous task of copyediting the manuscript—a job that required enormous patience on her part to deal with my request that "they" be used as a gender-neutral singular pronoun instead of the binary-reinforcing "him or her." I couldn't have asked for a more meticulous copyeditor.

A huge shout-out to the owner and staff of Grounded Coffee Shop in Alexandria, Virginia, for letting me loiter for five hours at a stretch, hunched over my laptop and sipping peppermint mochas, for three months straight.

Last but not least, I want to acknowledge the LGBTQ patients, families, and professionals who helped me realize the need for this book. Their journeys have not been easy ones. My hope is that the lessons we learn from their experiences with hospice and palliative care will help us ensure a smoother journey for those who come after them.

ABOUT LANGUAGE IN THIS BOOK

In writing *LGBTQ-Inclusive Hospice and Palliative Care,* I deliberately avoided opaque prose and used plain language instead. This is a scholarly work written to be accessible, practical, and understandable.

I use the term *LGBTQ* to be inclusive of all who self-identify as lesbian, gay, bisexual, transgender, gender non-conforming, queer, and/or questioning. (These terms are explained in Chapter 2 as well as in the Glossary.)

Throughout the text I alternate the order in which I use the terms hospice care and palliative care in recognition of the fact that the two aspects of the care continuum are equally important. Definitions for words and phrases that appear in bold type in the text can be found in the Glossary in the back of the book.

INTRODUCTION

FROM "SPECIAL POPULATION" TO INCLUSION — A PARADIGM SHIFT

When I began work on this book, I set out to write a resource for **hospice** and **palliative care** professionals that would be equally relevant and engaging to palliative care and hospice professionals from multiple disciplines; would change the way readers approach their work with *all* patients, not just with those who are lesbian, gay, bisexual, transgender, queer, and/or questioning (LGBTQ); and would show readers that having conservative religious or moral beliefs and providing high-quality, inclusive care to LGBTQ people and their families are not mutually exclusive. While the majority of the book is dedicated to achieving the first two goals, the third goal is equally important.

In the twelve years that I've been speaking to audiences about caring for LGBTQ individuals with chronic or life-limiting illnesses, one thing has remained fairly constant: health care providers with more conservative religious beliefs come to my presentations with significant discomfort at the outset — if they come at all. Changing the way LGBTQ individuals with chronic or life-limiting illnesses are cared for requires a paradigm shift in the way we (collectively, as health care professionals) approach the conversation about what it means to be inclusive in our compassion. You don't need to change your religious or moral beliefs to provide good care to LGBTQ individuals. So if you are unsure about buying or

Acquaviva, Kimberly
LGBTQ-Inclusive Hospice and Palliative Care
dx.doi.org/10.17312/harringtonparkpress/2017.03lgbtqihpc.00a
© 2017 by Kimberly Acquaviva

reading a book about LGBTQ people, don't be. At its core, this is simply a book about *people*.

LGBTQ-inclusive practice begins with an active choice—a choice to change our practice so that all are welcome and treated with dignity and compassion. I have never met a hospice or palliative care provider who consciously excludes LGBTQ individuals and their families. I do not believe that care professionals make a conscious choice to give poor care to LGBTQ individuals and their families. However, unless palliative care and hospice providers make a conscious choice to engage in LGBTQ-inclusive practice, they are, by default, unintentionally choosing to exclude LGBTQ people from receiving the high-quality care that all people deserve.

WHY THIS BOOK?

There is no shortage of well-researched publications for palliative care and hospice professionals. Several seminal works come to mind immediately:

- *Advanced Practice Palliative Nursing* (Dahlin, Coyne, and Ferrell 2016)
- *Dying in America: Improving Quality and Honoring Individual Preferences Near the End of Life* (Institute of Medicine 2015)
- *Geriatric Palliative Care* (Chai et al. 2014)
- *Oxford American Handbook of Hospice and Palliative Medicine and Supportive Care* (Yennurajalingam and Bruera 2016)
- *Oxford Textbook of Palliative Medicine* (Cherny et al. 2015)
- *Oxford Textbook of Palliative Nursing* (Ferrell, Coyle, and Paice 2015a)
- *Oxford Textbook of Palliative Social Work* (Altilio and Otis-Green 2011)
- *Pediatric Palliative Care* (Ferrell 2015)
- *Textbook of Palliative Care Communication* (Wittenberg et al. 2015)

In most of the texts listed, LGBTQ populations are either relegated to a stand-alone chapter, as is the case in the *Textbook of Palliative Care Communication* and the *Oxford Textbook of Palliative Social Work,* or they are mentioned briefly within the context of chapters on sexuality, "special populations," "cultural considerations," or HIV/AIDS, as in the *Oxford Textbook of Palliative Nursing,* the *Oxford Textbook of Palliative Medicine,* and *Geriatric Palliative Care.* There is no discussion at all of LGBTQ populations in *Pediatric Palliative Care,* with the exception of a brief mention in a chapter about **grief** and **bereavement** where the authors note that "single parents or same-sex parents may not have as many options for support as married parents in a heterosexual relationship" (Limbo and Davies 2015). *Advanced Practice Palliative Nursing* contains a brief acknowledgment that "the APRN will encounter a wide diversity of patients, such as military veterans; individuals with developmental disabilities; individuals with mental illness and personality disorders; prison inmates; the lesbian, gay, bisexual, transgender, and intersex community; individuals with substance use disorders; individuals who are homeless; and individuals of a low socioeconomic status" (Gibson 2016), but no content regarding how to provide LGBTQ-inclusive care. The most glaring absence of LGBTQ persons with serious or life-limiting illnesses, however, is in the 639-page *Dying in America: Improving Quality and Honoring Individual Preferences Near the End of Life,* in which the words and phrases *gay, lesbian, bisexual, transgender, sexual orientation, sexuality,* and *LGBTQ* are never used, not even once.

There is a critical need to move beyond ignoring the existence of LGBTQ people, thinking of LGBTQ people as a "special population," or conceptualizing LGBTQ people as a group that merits mention only within the context of discussions about disease and dysfunction. When LGBTQ people are relegated to a single chapter in a book, the clinicians most in need of the information may skip reading it entirely. Even more concerning, this approach to the presentation of content reinforces the idea that LGBTQ people are "other." (In *Advanced Practice Palliative Nursing,* the single mention of LGBTQ people is included in a list of other "special populations," sandwiched between "prison inmates" and "individuals with substance use disorders" [Gibson 2016]).

MAKING THE SHIFT TO LGBTQ-INCLUSIVE CARE

This book turns the traditional approach to addressing LGBTQ patients in palliative care and hospice upside down, in order to help clinicians make the shift from providing *special* care to LGBTQ people to instead providing *inclusive* care to *all* people, including those who are LGBTQ.

In writing *LGBTQ-Inclusive Hospice and Palliative Care,* I made a conscious decision to use a conversational tone rather than an academic one. Unlike discipline-specific books that cover dense, foundational content like the pathophysiology of pain, pharmacology, or pain and symptom management, this book seeks to provide both new and experienced hospice and palliative care professionals with the knowledge they need to shift from providing high-quality care to *high-quality LGBTQ-inclusive care.* You may be reading this and thinking that you already provide LGBTQ-inclusive care. You treat every person the same — why would your treatment of LGBTQ people and their families be any different? These are great questions, and ones I hear a lot. Providing LGBTQ-inclusive care requires a shift in the way you think about hospice and palliative care. Being inclusive is not the same as treating everyone the same. In fact, treating everyone the same is an approach that rarely benefits patients, regardless of whether they are LGBTQ, because patients aren't all the same. This book will give you clear, actionable strategies to use in transforming your care of patients so that it is truly LGBTQ-inclusive. The ultimate goal is for LGBTQ-inclusive care to be what you provide to *all* patients — not a "specialized" form of care provided to LGBTQ patients.

USING THIS BOOK TO MAKE THE SHIFT

Providing LGBTQ-inclusive hospice and palliative care involves making subtle changes in the way you approach almost every aspect of care. At first glance, the titles of chapters in this book may appear to reflect topics with which you are already quite familiar. While experienced hospice and palliative care professionals are likely to have a solid background in many of these broad topic areas, the chapters are designed to build on that knowledge rather than duplicate it. To get the maximum benefit out of this book, it is important to read all of the chapters. That being said, I have written this for readers in four distinct disciplines, medicine, nursing, chaplaincy, and social work/counseling, and your own discipline's **scope of practice** will determine whether and how you integrate the content into your professional practice. For example, although everyone should read the chapter on conducting a physical exam, if you are a chaplain, social worker, or counselor, you will not conduct physical exams yourself because they are outside your discipline's scope of practice.

Of course, you don't have to be a physician, registered nurse, advanced practice registered nurse, chaplain, social worker, or counselor to benefit from reading this book. Clinical psychologists, pharmacists, home health aides, licensed practical nurses, licensed massage therapists, registered dieticians, music therapists, speech-language pathologists, physical/rehabilitation therapists, volunteer coordinators, administrators, and educators, will find that this book can help change the way they work with patients, families, staff, students, and volunteers. And if you are a student, it will help you get off on the right foot in terms of LGBTQ-inclusive practice as you begin your work with patients and their families.

COMPETENCY-BASED SCAFFOLDING

LGBTQ-Inclusive Hospice and Palliative Care is built on a scaffolding of learning objectives designed to address the needs of physicians, advanced practice registered nurses

(APRNs), registered nurses (RNs), social workers, counselors, and chaplains working in the field of hospice and palliative care. I developed these learning objectives using discipline-specific competencies, curricular guidelines, and professional standards. Since there are no existing competencies focused on LGBTQ-inclusive hospice and palliative care, I set out to find and compile hospice and palliative care competencies first, and then LGBTQ-specific health care competencies. After gathering competencies in these two broad areas for the four target disciplines, I planned to create a crosswalk between the areas and develop working competencies for LGBTQ-inclusive hospice and palliative care for each discipline. At least, that was the original plan. I had mistakenly assumed it would be relatively easy to find hospice and palliative care competencies and LGBTQ-specific competencies for each of the disciplines, and that the challenge would be in converting them into LGBTQ-inclusive hospice and palliative care competencies.

Unfortunately, of the four health care disciplines this book addresses, only medicine has established detailed competencies for both the care of LGBTQ persons and the care of persons with chronic or life-limiting illnesses (see Association of American Medical Colleges [AAMC] 2014, American Academy of Hospice and Palliative Medicine [AAHPM] 2009, American Academy of Family Physicians [AAFP] n.d., Joint Commission 2011). The social work discipline has indicators for cultural **competence** and general standards for social work practice in palliative and hospice care but no set of competencies specific to working with LGBTQ individuals (National Association of Social Workers [NASW] 2007, NASW 2004, Hay and Johnson 2001). Similarly, the chaplaincy discipline has general competencies for hospice and palliative care chaplains but no competencies specific to working with LGBTQ people and their families (California State University Institute for Palliative Care and Healthcare Chaplaincy Network 2015).

In gathering palliative care and hospice competencies, I looked to the certification requirements outlined by the credentialing bodies in the four disciplines. The American Board of Medical Specialties administers the Hospice and Palliative Medicine (HPM) subspecialty for physicians, and the American Osteopathic Association's Bureau of Osteopathic Specialists administers the Certificate of Added Qualification (CAQ) in hospice and palliative medicine for osteopathic physicians. Certification requires completion of a fellowship as well as passage of a daylong examination (AAHPM n.d.).

The Hospice and Palliative Credentialing Center (HPCC) administers the Certified Hospice and Palliative Nurse credential as well as the Advanced Certified Hospice and Palliative Nurse credential. Certification requires completion of 500 hours of practice in the previous year (or 1,000 hours in the previous two years) as well as passage of a lengthy examination (HPCC 2016a, 2016b).

The Hospice Medical Director Certification Board (HMDCB) administers the Hospice Medical Director Certification, which requires "400 hours of broad hospice-related activities" and either "two years of work experience in a hospice setting during the previous 5 years," "current, valid board certification in hospice and palliative medicine through the American Board of Hospice and Palliative Medicine (ABHPM), the American Board of Medical Specialties (ABMS), or the American Osteopathic Association (AOA)," or "successful completion of a 12-month clinical hospice and palliative medicine training program accredited by the Accreditation Council for Graduate Medical Education (ACGME) or AOA" (HMDCB 2013).

The National Association of Social Workers Specialty Certification Program administers the Certified Hospice and Palliative Social Worker credential and the Advanced Certified Hospice and Palliative Social Worker credential. Certification requires several years of supervised practice as a hospice and palliative care social worker, but there is no examination.

The Board of Chaplaincy Certification administers the Certified Hospice and Palliative Care Chaplain credential.

Requirements for certification are substantial (including a ten-page essay, three years of experience in hospice and palliative care, and three recommendation letters), but no examination is required.

Because the medicine and nursing competencies were so detailed, I was able to compile a spreadsheet of the competencies from each of the disciplines and then develop working competencies appropriate to each discipline to fill in the gaps. This is not the best way to develop competencies, but it gave me a draft set around which to develop the content of the book. Perhaps *LGBTQ-Inclusive Hospice and Palliative Care* will stimulate leaders from the four disciplines to come together to develop competencies in LGBTQ-inclusive hospice and palliative care.

HOW THE BOOK IS ORGANIZED

Providing LGBTQ-inclusive hospice and palliative care requires changes at two levels: the individual and the institutional. At the individual level, hospice and palliative care professionals can shift toward providing more LGBTQ-inclusive care by adopting a structure of self-awareness and changing the way they assess, interact with, and support the patients and families they work with. At the institutional level, organizations can strengthen their inclusion of LGBTQ individuals and their families by (1) updating language on the forms they use, (2) developing LGBTQ-inclusive messages and outreach strategies, (3) hiring more LGBTQ staff, (4) offering equitable benefits to employees in same-gender relationships and transgender employees, and (5) providing training to employees and volunteers. The chapters in this book build on one another, starting from the individual level in Chapter 1 and working up to the institutional level in Chapter 10. The following is a brief overview.

Chapter 1 describes a seven-step process that hospice and palliative care professionals can use to improve their ability to provide inclusive, nonjudgmental care when planning, engaging in, and reflecting on a patient interaction. In addition, the chapter describes communication techniques as well as verbal and nonverbal approaches to facilitating LGBTQ-inclusive care.

Chapter 2 explains the relationships among sex, gender, gender identity, gender expression or gender presentation, gender discordance, gender nonconformity, gender dysphoria, sexual orientation, sexual behavior, sexuality, and sexual health and discusses their relevance in the palliative care and hospice setting. In addition, the chapter describes a two-step process for asking patients about their assigned birth sex and true gender and explains the use of gender-neutral pronouns.

Chapter 3 explains why, given the historical and contemporary contexts within which LGBTQ people live, it's not surprising that some LGBTQ patients and families may be reluctant to seek care. The chapter describes three kinds of barriers to palliative care and hospice care—perceptual, financial, and institutional—and offers a two-pronged approach to addressing such barriers for LGBTQ patients.

Chapter 4 describes a new LGBTQ-inclusive approach to taking a comprehensive history that places the primary emphasis on the patient as person.

Chapter 5 explains how to coordinate and facilitate a family meeting focused on shared decision making, how to use shared decision making for issues surrounding palliative sedation, and how family dynamics may play a role in the shared decision-making process.

Chapter 6 explains how to help patients and families identify their own unique goals for care, how to use a set of key questions to refocus interdisciplinary/interprofessional team meet-

Though I consider myself a conservative Christian, my eyes have been opened regarding the differences in moral and civil beliefs. Several years ago I cared for a patient who was a lesbian. As I made my visits and came to know her and the partner she had shared over twenty years of her life with, I realized that this couple was like any loving, committed couple that I had witnessed hundreds of times before. There were family photos throughout the home, children and grandchildren on both sides were involved, along with any number of relationship quirks that go along with a couple that has been together long-term. What grieved me the most about this experience was the fact that her partner . . . was unable to take Family and Medical Leave Act [FMLA] time because they weren't considered to be married. So as the patient continued to decline, her partner, with whom she had shared almost half of her life, continued to have to work six days a week, almost twelve hours a day, because she was unable to take time off.

Now, my own Christian beliefs still dictate to me that a marriage is solely between a man and a woman. However, I have come to the conclusion that any committed couple, who have been together a number of years, should have the same civil rights of those couples who are of opposite sex. The fact that my patient was a lesbian wasn't the eye-opener for me—it was the fact that as she lay dying, the love of her life was literally two blocks away, working, because she wasn't able to take FMLA time. This seemed very wrong to me. I hope you can use my experience. I have come to believe that though my Christian beliefs can be black-and-white, the bottom line for my faith is still "love," and those [who] love should be able to be by the side of those they love, no matter the gender of their partner.

—JENNIFER HAWKINS, RN, CHPN

ings on patient- and family-centered outcomes of care, and how to conduct an environmental and safety risk assessment.

Chapter 7 provides an overview of the ethical principles that guide practice, the elements of advance care planning, and the legal issues that may have an impact on LGBTQ individuals, in particular, as they navigate serious and life-threatening illness and seek to remain the authors of their own lives.

Chapter 8 provides specific, actionable strategies for teaching patients and families about patient-care skills, end-stage disease progression, pain and symptom management, medication management, disposal of supplies, and signs and symptoms of imminent death.

Chapter 9 explains the developmental tasks of life completion and life closure as well as the roles that despair, hope, and meaning play in the context of advanced illness. The chapter describes LGBTQ-inclusive assessment skills and supportive techniques for addressing psychosocial and spiritual issues, and explains how a spiritual/existential history and a spiritual/existential assessment differ. Finally, this chapter examines the ways in which the members of the interdisciplinary/ interprofessional team work in collaboration with one another to support the patient and family in achieving their goals for care in the psychosocial and spiritual/existential domains.

Chapter 10 explains how to assess the structural integrity of an institution's or program's bridge to LGBTQ individuals and their families, and how to construct that bridge in order to reach, welcome, and serve LGBTQ individuals and families. After you have finished reading Chapter 10, consider ways you can encourage your organization to implement the types of changes described.

Each chapter contains the following elements:

- **Chapter Objectives:** Actions or behaviors (e.g., list, describe, explain, recognize, discuss) you should be able to perform after reading the chapter.
- **Key Terms:** Words or phrases covered within the chapter and also defined in the Glossary at the back of the book.
- **Chapter Summary:** A brief overview of the chapter.
- **Perspectives:** Text boxes containing personal stories submitted by palliative care and hospice providers, patients, and families.
- **Key Points to Remember:** A list of the chapter's main ideas or takeaway points.
- **Discussion Questions:** Questions you can use for self-assessment or to guide team-based or classroom-based discussions about the chapter.
- **Chapter Activity:** An activity that provides an opportunity for applying or reflecting on the chapter's content.

At the back of the book, you will find a glossary of important terms, a list of the references cited, and brief biographies of the experts who reviewed and validated the content. Additional resources, such as downloadable pocket guides, can be found on the website for *LGBTQ-Inclusive Hospice and Palliative Care,* http://www.lgbtq-inclusive.com.

LGBTQ-INCLUSIVE HOSPICE AND PALLIATIVE CARE

CHAPTER 1

SELF-AWARENESS AND COMMUNICATION

CHAPTER OBJECTIVES

1. Recognize and assess your attitudes, beliefs, and feelings about sexual orientation, gender identity, and gender expression/gender presentation.

2. Recognize and assess your attitudes, beliefs, and feelings about the dying process and death.

3. Describe a three-step mitigation plan you can follow before each patient interaction to mitigate the power imbalance between patient and provider and prevent your attitudes and beliefs from having a negative impact on the care you provide.

4. List empathic and facilitating verbal and nonverbal behaviors you can use in delivering LGBTQ-inclusive care.

5. Explain how touch, humor, and self-disclosure can be either helpful or harmful to your relationship with a patient.

Key Terms: assumption, attitude, belief, CAMPERS, compassion, emotion, empathic behaviors, empathy, facilitating behaviors, humor, patient-centered, power imbalance, reflection, right to self-determination, self-awareness, self-disclosure, touch, unconscious bias

Acquaviva, Kimberly
LGBTQ-Inclusive Hospice and Palliative Care
dx.doi.org/10.17312/harringtonparkpress/2017.03lgbtqihpc.001
© 2017 by Kimberly Acquaviva

Providing inclusive care to patients with chronic or life-limiting illnesses requires self-awareness — an awareness of one's attitudes, beliefs, and emotions and the ways in which they shape interactions and patient care. For hospice and palliative care professionals, self-awareness should be an ongoing process rather than a static state of existence to strive toward. This chapter describes a seven-step process that hospice and palliative care professionals can follow to improve their ability to provide inclusive, nonjudgmental care when planning, engaging in, and reflecting on patient interactions. In addition, the chapter describes verbal and **nonverbal communication** techniques to facilitate LGBTQ-inclusive care.

SELF-AWARENESS

Being aware of your own **attitudes**, **beliefs**, and **emotions** and the ways in which they shape your interactions with patients and the care you provide is the first step toward providing inclusive care. This kind of insight entails **self-awareness** (Benbassat and Baumal 2005). For all health care professionals, including those in hospice and palliative care, self-awareness should be an ongoing process, not a static, ideal state of existence one strives toward. The following seven-step process can be used to improve your ability to provide inclusive, nonjudgmental care when you are planning, engaging in, and reflecting on a patient interaction. The mnemonic device for remembering the steps in this process is **CAMPERS**: clear purpose, attitudes and beliefs, mitigation plan, patient, emotions, reactions, and strategy.

STEP 1: KNOW YOUR CLEAR PURPOSE

As you approach an interaction with a patient, take a minute to think about the reason for that interaction. Every interaction has a purpose. Give conscious thought to identifying your *clear purpose* before the interaction, but keep in mind that your purpose may (and should) change during the interaction, based on the needs of the patient. Whether you're a physician, an advanced practice registered nurse (APRN), a registered nurse (RN), social worker, counselor, or chaplain, your purpose for an interaction with a patient will generally fall into one or more of the following categories:

- Provide supportive **presence**
- Gather information
- Transmit information
- Clarify understanding of information
- Collaborate to create a plan
- Administer a medication or treatment

STEP 2: KNOW YOUR ATTITUDES AND BELIEFS
As you approach any interaction with a patient or client, think about your *attitudes and beliefs* in relation to that person. If you are going to be meeting a new patient for the first time, pay attention to any **assumptions** you might be making based on information on the intake form or referral sheet.

Does the first or last name of the patient lead you to make assumptions about the race, ethnicity, religion, or cultural traditions of the patient? If so, how do these assumptions lead you to draw other conclusions about the patient—for example, what their home may look like, what their socioeconomic status is, what amount of family support they have, and so on? Take a look at the patient's address. What assumptions do you make based on the patient's zip code, or whether the address includes an apartment number? When you look at the referring diagnosis, what thoughts pop into your head? For example, if the diagnosis is lung cancer, do you instantly wonder whether the patient was a smoker? What about a diagnosis of cirrhosis — do you find yourself wondering whether the patient has a history of alcohol abuse? Does a diagnosis of HIV/AIDS make you wonder whether the patient is gay?

There is nothing wrong with having any of these thoughts. Human beings sort information based on patterns, prior experiences, and learned social norms. These prejudgments (prejudices) are instinctual, even though they are often inaccurate:

> We categorize, make assumptions, interpret, and infer from within a viewpoint we routinely use to advance our personal ends and desires. We are, in a word, naturally prejudiced in our favor. We reflexively and spontaneously gravitate to the slant on things that makes it easiest to gratify our desires and justify doing so, including the desire to be correct. We naturally shrink at the thought of being wrong, and conversely, delight in the thought of being right, and so often resist the attempts of others to "correct" us, especially when this involves beliefs that are fundamental and part of our personal identity. . . . When people act in accordance with the injunctions and taboos of the group to which they belong they naturally feel righteous. . . . Group norms are typically articulated in the language of morality and a socialized person inwardly experiences some sense of shame or guilt in violating a social taboo, and anger or moral outrage at others who do so. In other words, what commonly seems to be the inner voice of conscience is often nothing more than the internalized voice of social authority, the voice of our parents, our teachers, and other "superiors" speaking within us. (Paul and Adamson 1993)

When you find yourself wondering whether a patient "did something" to cause their illness, you are hearing what Paul and Adamson call the "internalized voice of social authority." You are subconsciously trying to make sense of the patient's illness by sorting the patient into the category of "other"—a category of taboo breakers from whom you feel comfortably distant, or perhaps uncomfortably close. When you subconsciously view a patient's illness through a lens of taboo and punishment, you may feel safe from experiencing a similar fate or fearful that a similar fate might befall you. In reality, of course, no one is "safe" from experiencing a life-limiting illness: nonsmokers get lung cancer, heterosexual people get HIV/AIDS, and nondrinkers get cirrhosis. The challenge for all of us as health care professionals and human beings is to become aware of our instinctual prejudgments and then counteract their ability to influence our decisions and behaviors.

If you are going to be seeing a patient you have met before, pay attention to your attitudes and beliefs about the patient. Do you find yourself dreading the visit because the patient is a hoarder or the house seems uncomfortably dirty to you? If the patient is wealthy and lives in a beautiful home, do you find yourself looking forward to that visit a little more than you look forward to others? Do you have more positive feelings about visits to a patient who is gay than visits to a patient who is straight (or vice versa)? Ask yourself the following questions, and be honest with yourself:

- Which patient do you feel more **compassion** for: a patient with lung cancer who smoked or a patient with lung cancer who never smoked?
- Which patient would you rather spend time visiting: a homeless patient who lives under a bridge or a patient who lives in a luxury high-rise apartment?
- Which patient would be harder for you to relate to: an evangelical Christian or a devout Muslim?
- Which patient would you rather have assigned to you: a gay man with rectal cancer or a heterosexual ("straight") woman with rectal cancer?
- Do you believe homosexuality is a sin?
- If you believe in heaven and hell, do you believe gay, lesbian, bisexual, and transgender people go to hell after they die?
- Do you feel as though it's "normal" for older people to die but not younger people?

An important part of this step is becoming more aware of your attitudes and beliefs about dying and death. Ask yourself these questions:

- How do you define a "good" death?
- When patients choose to go to the hospital to die because they don't want to die at home, do you silently think to yourself that this is a bad decision?
- What are your thoughts about the use of artificial nutrition and hydration at the end of life?
- When family members of a patient who is likely days from death insist that the patient be given artificial nutrition and hydration after you have clearly explained the risks, do you think to yourself that they are making the wrong decision and that they're "in denial"?
- When a palliative care patient decides not to pursue potentially life-extending or curative treatment, do you think to yourself that the patient has "given up"?
- When a patient has adult children who live nearby, work full-time, and say they cannot help with the patient's care, do you find yourself viewing those adult children negatively?

Thinking about these questions—and answering them honestly, even if the answers make you cringe a bit—will help you become more aware of your attitudes and beliefs. Without this self-awareness, you run the risk that an **unconscious bias** will play a detrimental role in your care of patients—an unconscious bias that can lead you to develop "stories" to fit your bias. For example, your bias could lead you to become judgmental and assume that a person living in subsidized housing is uneducated or living in an unsafe environment.

STEP 3: KNOW YOUR MITIGATION PLAN
The term *mitigation plan* is used in the business world to describe an aspect of risk management: "Mitigation plans eliminate the exposure of a business to risk, lessen the impact of a threat, or reduce the frequency or severity of risks. In order for mitigation to be effective, the risks must be identified ahead of time and a plan devised[,] ready for implementation[,] before or when the risk occurs" (Sandilands n.d.).

I worked as a social worker in hospice in South Dakota in the '90s and have such fond memories of the men [with HIV/AIDS] we worked with at the end of life, and their partners/families. While it was tragic and very sad to lose such a young, vibrant group of men, they taught me so much in my time with them. Those men taught me that quality of life is defined only by the person going through the illness. I saw a young man that we all felt had no quality of life due to his blindness, chronic diarrhea, pain, nausea, and [other] intractable symptoms but he, at his young age, saw being alive to be with his mother one more day as an acceptable quality of life for him. These men taught me the strength and bond of a homosexual relationship and what excellent caregivers men are to each other. At that time, there was no legal or binding arrangement for their relationships, but I witnessed unbelievable commitment to each other and a resiliency that was not always present in the heterosexual population that we served. I learned the value of humor in coping with very difficult times.

I think the most valuable lesson that I learned in my work with those gay men was other people's ability to adapt and overcome their apprehensions in working with this population. Parents who were not always comfortable with their sons' homosexuality were almost always able to allow love to overcome any barrier they had, and they provided wonderful, supportive care at the end of their sons' lives. I [have] worked with nurses who would refuse to take a homosexual patient with AIDS. One nurse overcame her apprehension and became the nurse to care for all the men on our caseload with AIDS. She grew to love serving her "boys" and became the greatest advocate for these men, their partners, and their families at the end of their lives. As treatment of AIDS changed, we began decreasing our hospice caseload of patients with AIDS and sometimes even discharged people with AIDS—a happy end to a very tragic time.

—LYNNE HUNTER, MSW

In the context of the CAMPERS self-awareness process, the term refers to the actions you plan to take to prevent the attitudes and beliefs identified in step 2 from having an impact on your interactions with a patient.

Your mitigation plan should also include actions you will take to minimize the **power imbalance** between you and the patient. A power imbalance exists when one person in a relationship has more authority, expertise, or access to resources than the other person. Patients receiving palliative care or hospice care are in a vulnerable position because they may be dependent on the health care professional for meeting some of their most basic human needs, such as relieving their pain, helping them perform their activities of daily living, and easing their emotional and spiritual distress.

Some of the phrases used by health care professionals exemplify the existence of this power imbalance. The terms *noncompliant, nonadherent,* and *in* **denial** are probably the best examples. These terms connote that a patient has failed to comply with, adhere to, or accept the care plan developed by a health care professional—and they imply that the patient's role in the relationship between provider and patient is to follow orders. But what does terminology like this say about our respect for a patient's **right to self-determination?** "Noncompliance" and "non-adherence" do not describe patients' failures—instead, they reflect our inability as health care professionals to help patients set goals they are motivated and able to achieve. The phrase "in denial" similarly reflects our inability as health care professionals to meet patients where they are and understand their perspective on their situation.

While most hospice and palliative care professionals have abandoned the use of terms like noncompliant in favor of more **patient-centered** terminology, there is still much work to be done at the individual level to mitigate the effects of attitudes and beliefs on the care provided. Your mitigation plan does not need to be complex. In fact, the best mitigation plans are so simple that they can be easily remembered and quickly implemented in less than a minute, before each interaction with a patient.

The following mitigation plan consists of three concrete steps—three questions and answers that, if you repeat them to yourself each time you meet with a patient, will help you mitigate the power imbalance between patient and provider and prevent your attitudes and beliefs from having a negative impact on the care you provide. I have used "I" statements so you can imagine how the plan could be used in your own practice.

- **Who is the story about?** The story is about the patient. What I believe and my own attitudes have nothing to do with the patient's story.
- **Who should be writing the story?** I am not writing this story. The patient should be the one writing the story. The patient is the author of the story throughout this illness and for the remainder of the patient's life.
- **What is my role?** My job is simply to give the patient the behind-the-scenes support needed to write the story. I won't try to tell the patient what to write or cast myself as a central character.

STEP 4: KNOW THE PATIENT
At this point, you have identified the purpose for your interaction with the patient, taken a look at your own attitudes, beliefs, and assumptions, and implemented a plan for miti-

gating both the patient-provider power differential and the impact of your attitudes and beliefs on the care you are going to provide. The fourth step in the self-awareness process is to know the *patient*. Knowing the patient goes beyond simply knowing their diagnosis and prognosis—you need to get to know who the patient is as a person and what is most important to them. The following list of questions can be asked when you first meet a patient, after a brief period of rapport-building conversation:

- What name do you use?
- What sex were you assigned at birth?
- What gender do you identify as now?
- What gender pronouns do you use? (e.g., he/him, she/her, them/their, ze/zir)
- What prompted your decision to seek palliative care or hospice care?
- Whom do you consider to be your "family"?
- To whom do you turn for support?
- What do you know about your diagnosis? Prognosis?
- What are your short-term and longer-term goals for your life? For your care?

While several of these questions are standard components of a palliative care or hospice admission visit, the three questions about sex, gender, and gender pronouns may be unfamiliar to you. *These questions should be asked of all patients—not just those you think may be transgender.* The questions are discussed in greater depth in Chapter 2.

STEP 5: KNOW YOUR EMOTIONS

The fifth step in the self-awareness process is to learn to recognize your *emotions*. I still remember one of the first deaths I witnessed as a new social worker. Shortly after the patient took his last breath, I felt my eyes well up with tears and a lump form in my throat. When I glanced over at the patient's

I think a really good place to start in caring for the LGBT community is to get on the same page with patients and clients about language (i.e., personal pronouns, words for "partner," etc.). If you don't know, ask! It's OK to show that you don't know, because asking shows you care to get it right. Once you are informed, either directly or indirectly, it's so important to apply what you've learned about the language that people prefer. I once was involved with a situation where a hospice professional, Mr. A., gave a report referring to the male partner of a male patient as his "wife." That seemed unusual to the rest of us on the team because the male partner had clearly identified himself as the patient's husband in his interactions with us. When I asked Mr. A. about it, he said he was told by the male partner to refer to him as the patient's wife. When we sought clarification from the patient's husband about his preferred language, he reiterated that he is the patient's husband. The patient's husband reported that when he told Mr. A. that he was the patient's husband, Mr. A. continued to question it and didn't seem to "get it." The patient's husband finally [gave up and] told Mr. A., "Just think of me as [the patient's] wife." As a community, let's not be dense—let's ask for patient and family preferences and let's honor them!

—VICKI QUINTANA, RN, BSN

wife, though, her eyes were dry and I thought she looked almost bored. I felt a flicker of disapproval. I had *just* met the man and I was tearful. The word "cold" popped into my mind, followed by a cheek-burning sense of shame that in a split second I had unconsciously imposed my idea of what grief looks like onto her. Recognizing my emotions made it possible for me to move past them and focus on the emotions of the patient's wife. I sat with her and reminded myself that I needed to meet her where she was. Recognizing my emotions made it possible for me to put my feelings aside so that I could focus on the feelings that really mattered—those of the patient and his family.

As hospice and palliative care professionals, it can be difficult for us to acknowledge experiencing socially undesirable emotions. How often have you heard a patient, family member, friend, or neighbor say that you're an "angel" or a "saint" for the work that you do? It can be tough to reconcile the way that others see you (and the way you want to be seen) with the gritty emotions you experience working with patients and families. The fastest way to shed this sense of cognitive dissonance is to accept the fact you are not and cannot be a saint or an angel. You are a mortal human being doing incredibly challenging work to make the lives of patients and families better during illness, death, and bereavement. Feeling frustration or disgust or annoyance with patients doesn't mean you're a "bad" health care professional—it means you are human. Your task is to do whatever you can to recognize those feelings when you experience them and then make a conscious choice not to let them get in the way of your ability to provide the best care possible to patients.

STEP 6: KNOW YOUR REACTIONS

The sixth step in the self-awareness process, know your *reactions,* is closely intertwined with step 5. When you feel annoyance, do you convey that reaction to others in your facial expressions, body language, and tone of voice? Do you furrow your brow or maybe wrinkle your nose? What about when you feel frustrated with someone? Your goal in step 6 is to gain a better understanding of how your reactions become visible to others so you can make a conscious effort to avoid communicating those personal feelings to patients. One of the medical students I taught years ago would twirl her hair with her finger and bounce her foot up and down, dangling her shoe from her toes, when she was feeling a lack of confidence during an interaction with a patient. Once she was aware of both what she was feeling and her reaction to it, she was able to stop bouncing her foot and playing with her hair and begin projecting more confidence. Another medical student would register shock or surprise by widening her eyes and raising her eyebrows. She worked hard to control her facial expressions and is now a skilled practitioner with a rock-solid yet compassionate poker face.

If you are not sure how you show your emotions, ask your partner or spouse, family members, or friends. Ask them how they can tell when you are annoyed, frustrated, angry, disapproving, or impatient. The insights you glean will help you put this step into practice, so that when you are interacting with a patient and you recognize that you're experiencing an emotion you would rather not make visible to them, you can make a conscious effort to control your "tells"—the physical reactions, like pursed lips, furrowed brows, or crossed arms, that reveal your feelings.

STEP 7: KNOW YOUR STRATEGY

The last step in the self-awareness process is know your *strategy*. This step involves taking time for a brief period of review after an interaction with a patient, in order to develop a strategy for communicating more effectively in future interactions. Think about what went well in your interaction and what did not. Were you surprised by any of the thoughts or emotions you experienced during the interaction? How did those emotions make themselves visible to the patient? Were you able to support the patient's role as the author of their own story, or did you find yourself trying to take control of that story at times? Whose goals and needs were met during the interaction—the patient's, yours, both? Based on how the interaction went, consider what you would do differently or better in your next patient interaction, and devise a strategy for carrying this out in the future.

COMMUNICATION

The CAMPERS process—clear purpose, attitudes and beliefs, mitigation plan, patient, emotions, reactions, and strategy— when paired with good communication skills, will help you provide inclusive, nonjudgmental care. Communicating with patients and their families is central to your work as a hospice or palliative care professional. APRNs, RNs, physicians, chaplains, social workers, and counselors learn communication skills in school, with each discipline putting a unique spin on the communication techniques that are taught. Because the focus of this book is on the skills hospice and palliative professionals need to deliver LGBTQ-inclusive care, I will not be covering basic communication skills. Instead, this book will highlight communication techniques and other verbal and nonverbal approaches that facilitate LGBTQ-inclusive care.

Empathic behaviors are the things you say (verbal) or do (nonverbal) to convey to patients that you care about them and are committed to understanding their perspective or experience, and **facilitating behaviors** are the things you say or do to foster open communication (AAHPM 2009). Table 1.1 summarizes the behaviors.

The behaviors listed in table 1.1 can convey **empathy** and facilitate open communication, but if carried out clumsily or insincerely, some of these behaviors can be detrimental to forming a relationship with a patient, especially when it comes to being LGBTQ-inclusive. Three behaviors in particular are open to misuse by well-meaning professionals: **self-disclosure**, **touch**, and **humor**.

SELF-DISCLOSURE

Disclosing information about yourself can convey empathy and openness, but the disclosure should be made to meet

TABLE 1.1 EMPATHIC AND FACILITATING BEHAVIORS

	VERBAL	NONVERBAL
Empathic	silence listening affirmation self-disclosure	touch open posture facial expression
Facilitating	naming normalization reflection humor	eye contact head nodding/shaking eye-level approach

Source: AAHPM 2009. Reprinted with permission from the American Academy of Hospice and Palliative Medicine, © 2009 American Academy of Hospice and Palliative Medicine.

the needs of the patient, not those of the health care professional (you). If you self-identify as lesbian, gay, bisexual, transgender, gender nonconforming, queer, and/or questioning, you may find yourself wanting to share this fact with the LGBTQ patients you work with. Before you do, think about your rationale for disclosing this information. Would you be doing it because you want the patient to like you? Trust you? Feel understood by you? Are there other ways you could accomplish those goals more effectively? The same questions hold true for heterosexual hospice and palliative care professionals. If you self-identify as heterosexual and you find yourself wanting to mention your other-gender significant other or spouse during a conversation with a patient, think carefully about your rationale for doing so. Why do you want to disclose your heterosexuality? Whose needs are you meeting— yours or the patient's? Self-disclosure is neither good nor bad. Use it with intentionality to maximize its potential benefits.

There are ways other than verbal self-disclosure to show that you are committed to providing nonjudgmental care to LGBTQ individuals and their families. Some providers wear a rainbow "ally" lapel pin as a way to signal to patients and families that they are committed to LGBTQ-inclusive care.

AUTHOR'S NOTE

Over the years I've been asked many times why lesbian, gay, and bisexual people feel the need to "tell people about their sex lives" by coming out to others. Rather than answer the question directly, I like to respond by asking the questioner to try the following exercise. If you are heterosexual and currently in a relationship with a person of the other gender, keep track of how many times you make reference to this person (either by name or by such terms as boyfriend, girlfriend, husband, wife) in your conversations with colleagues, friends, neighbors, and family members this week. At the end of the week, reflect on why you felt the need to share your heterosexuality with so many people.

This exercise never fails to leave people surprised by how often heterosexuality is casually disclosed in everyday conversations. Mentioning your sexual orientation to others isn't telling people about your sex life; it is sharing a part of who you are as a person.

TOUCH

When touch is a part of care delivery — for example, when a nurse puts lotion on a patient's dry skin or a chaplain holds hands with a patient in prayer — it can be a powerful tool for conveying a sense of caring and compassion. When touch is used during a conversation between a professional and a patient, however, it can be awkward. Does putting a hand on a patient's knee make potentially difficult news easier to hear, or does it just make us as professionals think we are doing something to lessen the patient's pain? As a social worker and as a patient, I view touch as something that needs to be invited. I do not want my health care providers to pat me on the knee or rub my back, and I don't do those things to patients I work with. Touch may even be physically or emotionally painful for a patient, so refrain from touching without a patient's invitation and consent. Each patient you work with will have different preferences in terms of touch; it is important to be cognizant of that.

Hugging is particularly tricky territory. A patient who has a history of sexual abuse, for example, may feel triggered by a forced or unexpected embrace. The power differential between the hospice and palliative care professional and the patient may make it difficult for the patient to refuse a hug initiated by a care provider. Talk with all of your patients about touch and ask them about their desire for and level of comfort with hugs from you. This may seem like a small thing, but the importance of respecting patients' physical and emotional boundaries cannot be overstated.

HUMOR

Like touch, humor is a behavior that should be used carefully and with an awareness of the needs and preferences of each patient. A joking comment that seems lighthearted to you may seem callous to a patient or family member. A patient with a chronic or life-limiting illness — especially a patient in physical pain — may not appreciate your attempts at humor. This is not to say that there is no place for laughter in hospice or palliative care — on the contrary, laughter has many physiological and psychological benefits (Mayo Foundation for Medical Education and Research n.d.b).

There are different ways to use humor, including laughing at oneself, laughing at the other person, laughing at a situation, and laughing at someone other than the two people interacting. Within the context of your relationship with a patient, it is wise to avoid laughing at the patient or laughing at someone else. This kind of humor runs the risk of being interpreted as mean-spirited and hurtful. Laughing at the absurdity of a situation is safer territory, especially if the patient initiates the laughter.

When I was twenty-six, I was finishing up my dissertation proposal at my childhood home in Texas while caring for my mom, who was dying of ovarian cancer. The morning of the day she died, friends and family members were gathered around her on her bed, telling funny stories and sharing memories. She was minimally responsive—it was clear to all of us that she would die within hours. Suddenly she smiled slightly and said, "You know, I'm not dead yet." Our laughter at her parting joke ended up sweetening all our tears. Had a hospice professional cracked the joke, saying, "You know, she's not dead yet," it wouldn't have been funny at all—it would have come across as cruel. Remember that humor relies on context as much as content.

KEY POINTS TO REMEMBER

- CAMPERS is a seven-step process you can use to improve your ability to provide inclusive, nonjudgmental care when you are planning, engaging in, and reflecting on a patient interaction. The letters in the mnemonic device stand for: clear purpose, attitudes and beliefs, mitigation plan, patient, emotions, reactions, and strategy.
- Every interaction with a patient should have a clear purpose. Give conscious thought to your purpose before an interaction, but keep in mind that your purpose may (and should) change based on the needs of the patient during the interaction.
- As you approach an interaction with a patient, take a minute to think about your attitudes and beliefs in relation to that patient. Become aware of any prejudgments so that you can counteract the ability of those judgments to influence your decisions and behaviors.
- Review your mitigation plan before each patient interaction as a reminder to mitigate the power imbalance between patient and provider and prevent your attitudes

and beliefs from having a negative impact on the care you provide.

- Get to know who the patient is as a person and what is most important to the patient.

- Recognize your own emotions during your interactions with patients and make a conscious choice not to let them get in the way of your ability to provide the best care possible.

- Avoid making your emotional reactions visible when interacting with a patient. When you recognize that you are experiencing an emotion you would rather not communicate, make a conscious effort to control your "tells" (e.g., pursed lips, furrowed brows, crossed arms).

- Engage in a brief period of review after each interaction with a patient so that you can develop a strategy for communicating more effectively in the future.

DISCUSSION QUESTIONS

1. Why is it important to recognize and assess your attitudes, beliefs, and feelings about sexual orientation, gender identity, and gender expression or gender presentation in order to provide LGBTQ-inclusive care? Can you provide LGBTQ-inclusive care *without* this self-awareness? Why or why not?

2. Growing up, what messages did you hear regarding sexual orientation, gender identity, and gender expression or gender presentation? How did these messages shape the attitudes, beliefs, and feelings you have today?

3. Imagine you have been asked to care for an LGBTQ patient. Describe how you would use the CAMPERS self-awareness process before, during, and after your first interaction with the patient.

4. Describe how you might use verbal and nonverbal techniques to convey empathy and facilitate communication with a patient who seems reluctant to talk openly with you.

5. Imagine that you are meeting with a new patient recently diagnosed with the same rare, life-threatening illness that your close friend had, who was treated and cured. The patient is sobbing and you want to offer some comfort. Give examples of how touch, humor, and self-disclosure might be used *inappropriately* in this scenario.

CHAPTER ACTIVITY

Use the CAMPERS self-awareness process before, during, and after an interaction with a patient (either a real interaction or one simulated via role playing). Immediately afterward, write down what you were thinking and feeling during each step in the process. Did any of your thoughts or feelings surprise you? If you used the CAMPERS process for your work with all patients, do you think it would decrease the impact of unconscious bias on the care you deliver? Why or why not?

CHAPTER 2

SEX, GENDER, SEXUAL ORIENTATION, BEHAVIOR, AND HEALTH

CHAPTER OBJECTIVES

1. Define sex and gender and describe the differences between them.
2. Define gender identity and gender expression or gender presentation and describe the differences between them.
3. Define gender discordance, gender nonconformity, and gender dysphoria and describe how they differ.
4. Define sexual orientation and sexual behavior and describe the differences between them.
5. Define sexuality and sexual health.

Key Terms: asexual, bisexual, cisgender, gay, gender, gender discordance, gender dysphoria, gender expression, gender identity, gender nonconformity, gender presentation, heterosexual, homosexual, lesbian, pansexual, sex, sexual behavior, sexual expression, sexual health, sexuality, sexual orientation, transgender

Acquaviva, Kimberly
LGBTQ-Inclusive Hospice and Palliative Care
dx.doi.org/10.17312/harringtonparkpress/2017.03lgbtqihpc.002
© 2017 by Kimberly Acquaviva

Providing LGBTQ-inclusive care requires an understanding of several key concepts: sex, gender, gender identity, gender expression or presentation, gender discordance, gender nonconformity, gender dysphoria, sexual orientation, sexual behavior, sexuality, and sexual health. This chapter explains how these concepts relate to one another and their relevance in the palliative care and hospice setting. In addition, the chapter describes a two-step process for asking patients about their assigned birth sex and true gender and explains the use of gender-neutral pronouns.

KNOWLEDGE DEFICITS

When I teach, I never cease to be amazed by the number of health-professions students who lack basic knowledge about human sexuality. Without exception, these are bright students who graduated from good undergraduate programs. With a recent group of graduate students, I gave out a questionnaire so that I could build the weekly course content around their knowledge gaps. I asked them to submit the questions they've always wanted to ask about human sexuality. Questions that the students submitted included the following (reproduced here verbatim):

- "Has being gay become a fad more than an actual identity that one is born with? Do you think some people just give up on the opposite sex or somewhere along the way, they become influenced by friends?"
- "Can someone really be born gay/lesbian?"
- "I have always wondered whether being a gay is a 'social disease'/trend or is it really genetic?"
- "Is it truly possible to be bisexual?"
- "I don't understand transgendered people and I don't know how to gracefully have a conversation with some- one who is transgendered without being inquisitive or trying to satisfy my own curiosity about their lifestyle."

To address the knowledge deficits related to human sexuality that seem to be fairly common among health care professionals, this chapter provides a quick overview of the key concepts you need to understand in order to provide good care to all patients, including those who are LGBTQ. For a more in-depth exploration of some of these concepts, check out Nicholas Teich's book *Transgender 101: A Simple Guide to a Complex Issue* (2012) and Laura Erickson-Schroth's *Trans Bodies, Trans Selves: A Resource for the Transgender Community* (2014).

SEX AND GENDER

Two words that you may have heard used interchangeably are **sex** and **gender**. Sex has to do with biology and physiology and gender has to do with sociocultural expectations, roles, and behaviors (Gendered Innovations n.d.). When a baby is born and the clinician says, "Congratulations, it's a girl!" this observation of the baby's sex is based on the appearance of the genitals.

The X and Y chromosomes determine sex, with most human females having a 46XX chromosomal makeup and most males having a 46XY chromosomal makeup. The role of chromosomes in determining sex is not always that clear-cut, however. Babies may be born with sex monosomies (46X or 46Y, missing an X chromosome) or sex polysomies (46XXX, 46XXY, and so on), or with translocations of portions of their chromosomes (resulting in a male with 46XX or a female with 46XY) (WHO 2016b). Babies may also be born with what is known as an intersex condition with simple or complex variance. Sex can be described as a continuum that has male and female as its two endpoints. Between those two points, the science is imprecise:

> Nature presents us with sex anatomy spectrums. . . . [S]ex categories get simplified into male, female, and sometimes intersex, in order to simplify social interactions, express what

we know and feel, and maintain order. So nature doesn't decide where the category of "male" ends and the category of "intersex" begins, or where the category of "intersex" ends and the category of "female" begins. Humans decide. Humans (today, typically doctors) decide how small a penis has to be, or how unusual a combination of parts has to be, before it counts as intersex. Humans decide whether a person with XXY chromosomes or XY chromosomes and androgen insensitivity will count as intersex. (Intersex Society of North America 2008)

Gender is a social construct that varies across geography, culture, and time. While sex is about the physical body of a person, gender is about the way the person inhabiting that physical body feels, behaves, and is "read" by the society around them. If gender expression were described as a continuum, its endpoints would be masculine and feminine.

GENDER IDENTITY AND EXPRESSION OR PRESENTATION

An individual's **gender identity** refers to that person's internal sense of being a man or a woman. **Gender expression**, or **gender presentation**, is the way a person outwardly expresses that internal sense. When I speak to groups of health professionals, I often use myself as an example to illustrate the concept of gender identity and gender expression. I was born into a female body and was assigned the sex "female" at birth. My internal sense of myself is that I am a woman, and I self-identify as feminine. My gender identity is that of a woman.

When their gender identity aligns with the sex they were assigned at birth, individuals may refer to themselves as **cisgender**, or "cis." For example, let's say Bob was assigned the sex "male" at birth. Bob identifies as a man and presents himself to the world as a man. Bob might use the term *cisgender* to describe himself. The term *cisgender* has both enthusiastic proponents and critics. Some argue that it perpetuates a binary way of seeing the world as either "us" or "them" (White 2013).

Indeed, the Latin prefix *cis-* means "on this side of," while the prefix *trans-* means "on the other side of" (Steinmetz 2014). Others argue the term is simply a descriptor.

AUTHOR'S NOTE

I express my gender identity (my internal sense of my gender and, more broadly, my core sense of being) through the way I present my physical self to the world. When I step outside my home, I feel as though I'm walking out into the world presenting myself as a woman. Sometimes I wear lipstick and earrings and high heels, sometimes I wear jeans, flannel shirts, and Doc Martens. But always, no matter what clothing I wear, I am presenting myself to the world as a woman.

As a woman with very short hair who has had an unreconstructed prophylactic bilateral mastectomy, however, I may be "read" by other people as masculine looking. My gender identity as a woman is unwavering, but how others see my gender may not match how I see myself. Does my flat chest make me a man? Of course not. The absence or presence of breasts has nothing to do with whether a person is female. So whose opinion counts when it comes to determining how to interpret my gender expression or gender presentation — mine or that of the person viewing me? Mine.

That's why you should never attempt to make a visual determination of a patient's sex, gender identity, or gender expression. Instead, ask. The patient will tell you what you need to know in order to provide the best care.

GENDER DISCORDANCE, GENDER NONCONFORMITY, AND GENDER DYSPHORIA

The word *conformity* is generally used in reference to an external set of rules or expectations. **Gender nonconformity** describes behavior (including appearance and choice of clothing) that fails to conform to socially constructed norms or expectations (Adelson and Bockting 2014). When a child is assigned the male sex at birth, for example, and from a very

Some people use pronouns other than the gendered pronouns *he* and *she* to describe themselves. A person may feel constrained by gendered (sometimes called "binary") pronouns for any number of reasons. It doesn't mean the person self-identifies as LGBTQ. For this reason, at your first meeting you should ask about the gender pronouns an individual uses. This practice helps to facilitate patient-centered care and communication (National LGBT Health Education Center 2015). If you're not sure how to ask about the pronouns a person uses, here's an example of a good way to start: "I'm Mark and I like to be referred to with the pronouns *he, him,* and *his*. What pronouns do you use?" In the following chart the gendered pronouns *she* and *he* are followed by just a few of the gender-neutral pronouns you might hear once you begin asking people about their preferences.

Gender Pronouns

Please note that these are not the only pronouns. There are an infinite number of pronouns as new ones emerge in our language. Always ask someone for their pronouns.

Subjective	Objective	Possessive	Reflexive	Example
she	her	hers	herself	She is speaking. I listened to her. The backpack is hers.
he	him	his	himself	He is speaking. I listened to him. The backpack is his.
they	them	theirs	themself	They are speaking. I listened to them. The backpack is theirs.
ze	hir/zir	hirs/zirs	hirself/zirself	Ze is speaking. I listened to hir. The backpack is zirs.

Source: Chart © Landyn Pan (Trans Student Educational Resources 2016). Reprinted with permission.

young age insists on wearing only dresses, that child may be described as exhibiting gender nonconforming behavior. Similarly, my flat chest and short hair may be viewed by some people as examples of gender nonconformity. Gender nonconformity is defined by the viewer, in contrast to gender discordance and gender dysphoria, both of which rely on an individual's internal perceptions of their own gender. When a person's anatomical sex doesn't match their gender identity, this is referred to as **gender discordance**. For example, a person with gender discordance may be assigned a female sex at birth and identify as male, but not experience any distress over this. When the person is distressed over this mismatch, it is referred to as **gender dysphoria** (Adelson and Bockting 2014).

Some individuals whose anatomical sex doesn't match their gender identity choose to take steps to bring their gender expression or gender presentation into alignment with their gender identity. These individuals may describe themselves using terms like **transgender** or **genderqueer**, or they may reject such labels and simply describe themselves using the term that best aligns with their gender identity. Some individuals choose to dress and groom themselves (e.g., through shaving, hairstyle, makeup) in a way that outwardly reflects their internal gender identity, while leaving their physical body as it is. Other individuals choose to make modifications to their physical body, using hormones, hormone blockers, surgery, or a combination of treatments. When you are working with a patient whose assigned sex at birth does not match the patient's true gender identity, don't assume that the patient has had (or wants to have) surgery to align their anatomy with their identity. There is no right or wrong way for people to bring their gender expression or gender presentation into alignment with their gender identity, and not everyone chooses to do so at all. Gender identity is completely distinct from sexual orientation: a person may be transgender and heterosexual. For example, a person assigned the male sex at birth who currently identifies as female might describe herself as heterosexual if she were attracted primarily or solely to men.

MAKING SENSE OF COMPLEXITY

So if sex is determined by biology and physiology, and gender identity depends on how an individual self-identifies, what can you infer about a person's birth sex and gender identity based on the fact that the person checked "male" rather than "female" on an intake form? Unfortunately, the information collected from this patient is useless. Did the patient check "male" because they are biologically and physiologically male or because their gender identity is male? There is no way you can know what the patient meant by the answer. This is a common problem with traditional intake and admission forms—a problem that can be compounded when health care professionals check the boxes on the form themselves without even asking the patient the questions.

Sometimes clinicians will modify their forms in an attempt to be inclusive, only to miss the mark. If you ask patients to identify themselves as "male," "female," "transgender," or "other," you run the risk of missing "some transgender people who do not identify as such (e.g., a person who was born male, but whose gender identity is female, may check 'female' rather than 'transgender' on a form)" (National LGBT Health Education Center 2015).

To gather relevant clinical information about sex and gender from all patients, you need to ask patients two questions at the time of their intake: (1) What sex were you assigned at birth? (2) What gender do you identify as now?

These questions should be asked of all patients, not just those you think might be transgender (Fenway Institute and the Center for American Progress 2014, Institute of Medicine 2011, Joint Commission 2011). If these two questions are asked at intake, they should not have to be repeated multiple times by different members of the team.

The two-step method of asking patients about both birth sex and gender identity has been found to yield more complete data, and the Centers for Disease Control asserts that "using the two-step data collection method of asking for sex assigned at birth and current gender identity can help to increase the likelihood that transgender people will be accurately identified" (Tate, Ledbetter, and Youssef 2013; Centers for Disease Control 2016). In a study involving four health centers with diverse patient populations, the overwhelming majority of participants understood the questions in the two-step method, and "eighty-five percent strongly agreed that they would answer the birth sex question, and 78 percent strongly agreed that they would answer the current gender identity question" (Fenway Institute and the Center for American Progress 2014).

If a patient's anatomical sex at birth does not match their gender identity, you can follow up by asking, "What pharmacological or surgical steps, if any, have you taken in the past to bring your gender expression or presentation into alignment with your gender identity?" It may be helpful to explain that this information is important for you to know as the health care provider, so that you and the patient can work in partnership to plan the most appropriate care moving forward.

SEXUAL ORIENTATION AND SEXUAL BEHAVIOR

The American Psychological Association defines **sexual orientation** broadly to include attraction, identity, behavior, and community membership: "Sexual orientation refers to an enduring pattern of emotional, romantic, and/or sexual attractions to men, women, or both sexes. Sexual orientation also refers to a person's sense of identity based on those attractions, related behaviors, and membership in a community of others who share those attractions" (American Psychological Association 2008). While sexual orientation *may* refer to all of these components, in clinical practice the term is most commonly used to refer to the first sentence of the American

Psychological Association's definition. For the purposes of this book, sexual orientation refers to a person's sexual, emotional, and/or relational attraction to men, women, or both.

A **heterosexual** woman is primarily attracted to men, and a heterosexual man is primarily attracted to women; both are commonly referred to as "straight." A woman whose sexual orientation is **homosexual (lesbian** or **"gay")** is primarily attracted to women. A man whose sexual orientation is homosexual (gay) is primarily attracted to men. A man or woman whose sexual orientation is **bisexual** is attracted to both men and women and is commonly referred to as "bi." (Individuals who are attracted to a combination of genders may self-identify as **pansexual**). The only way to determine a person's sexual orientation is to ask—sexual orientation can't be inferred from observed or even self-reported sexual behavior. Some individuals do not identify as having sexual, emotional, or relational attractions to anyone. These individuals may refer to themselves as **asexual**.

Sexual behavior refers to acts engaged in by an individual toward the goal of sexual pleasure, reproduction, or both. Sexual behavior can involve a wide range of activities: oral-genital, oral-oral, genital-genital, oral-anal, genital-anal, manual-anal, and manual-genital contact are just a few of the ways that individuals may engage in sexual behavior with another person. Sexual behavior also need not involve another person—masturbation, or self-stimulation, is considered sexual behavior as well.

Sexual expression is a term used to describe the way in which individuals express their sexual desires, either alone or with partners. It is more than "sex": "Sexual expression is a form of communication through which we give and receive pleasure and emotion. It has a wide range of possibilities—from sharing fun activities, feelings and thoughts, warm touch or hugs, to physical intimacy. It is expressed both individually and in relationships throughout life" (McKinley Health Center 2009).

As a bisexual it's incredibly difficult to be out. Because unless you tell them, there is no way they're going to guess. You know, if you're seen with a same sex partner you're judged to be a lesbian; if you're seen with the opposite sex partner you're judged to be straight. Or you might be by yourself and is it relevant to say anything? You're constantly passing for what you're not, and it's really frustrating.

—KATHRYN ALMACK, PHD

From *The Last Outing: Exploring End of Life Experiences and Care Needs in the Lives of Older LGBT People* (Almack et al. 2014).

SEXUALITY AND SEXUAL HEALTH

To understand the concept of sexual health, an understanding of a more foundational concept—**sexuality**—is needed. The World Health Organization defines sexuality as: "A central aspect of being human throughout life [that] encompasses sex, gender identities and roles, sexual orientation, eroticism, pleasure, intimacy and reproduction. Sexuality is experienced and expressed in thoughts, fantasies, desires, beliefs, attitudes, values, behaviors, practices, roles and relationships. While sexuality can include all of these dimensions, not all of them are always experienced or expressed. Sexuality is influenced by the interaction of biological, psychological, social, economic, political, cultural, legal, historical, religious and spiritual factors" (WHO 2006, 2010).

What's notable about this definition is that it asserts that sexuality is "a central aspect of being human throughout life." Whether the patient is thirty years old or ninety, sexuality is a central aspect of that patient's humanity. The same is true for the patient who is weeks or days from death: sexuality remains central to their being: "Even patients facing terminal illness may desire to remain sexually active if possible. This needs to be placed within the overall context of goals and desires for care. Patients and their loved ones may feel uncomfortable initiating discussion about sexuality and sexual health needs in the context of palliative care. In most cultures, sexuality, significant illness, and dying are all considered taboo topics, at least to some degree, so it becomes part of the healthcare professional's duty to raise these issues" (Griebling 2016).

If sexuality is a central part of being human throughout the lifespan, what does it mean for a patient in palliative care or hospice care to experience sexual health? The World Health Organization declares that **sexual health** is "a state of physical, emotional, mental and social well-being in relation to sexuality[;] it is not merely the absence of disease, dysfunction or infirmity. Sexual health requires a positive and respectful approach to sexuality and sexual relationships, as well as the possibility of having pleasurable and safe sexual experiences, free of coercion, discrimination and violence. For sexual health to be attained and maintained, the sexual rights of all persons must be respected, protected and fulfilled" (WHO 2006, 2010).

Patients in palliative care and hospice care can experience sexual health. While sexual health "is not merely the absence of disease, dysfunction or infirmity," the presence of disease, dysfunction, or infirmity does not negate the possibility for a patient of experiencing sexual health.

In its *Clinical Practice Guidelines for Quality Palliative Care*, the National Consensus Project for Quality Palliative Care highlights the importance of sexual health by including it in the criteria that need to be addressed. In determining the social aspects of patient care, according to Guideline 4.2 the palliative care team should conduct "a comprehensive, person-centered, interdisciplinary assessment" of the social needs and goals of each patient and family, including:

"Strengths and vulnerabilities: resiliency; social and cultural support networks; effects of illness or injury on intimacy and sexual expression; prior experiences with illness, disability, and loss; risk of abuse, neglect, or exploitation" (National Consensus Project for Quality Palliative Care 2013; Altilio, Otis-Green, and Dahlin 2008).

Sexual health is as achievable and reasonable a goal for patients in palliative care and hospice care as pain relief, but few hospice and palliative care professionals include sexual health within their assessment and plan of care. Given that sexuality is a central aspect of being human, sexual health should be part of the assessment and plan for every patient receiving palliative care and hospice care. Chapter 4 explains how to incorporate sexual health into the assessment process, and Chapter 6 provides specific suggestions for how to incorporate sexual health into a patient's palliative or hospice care plan.

KEY POINTS TO REMEMBER

- *Sex* has to do with the biology and physiology of being male or female. *Gender* has to do with the sociocultural expectations, roles, and behaviors of men and women.
- While sex refers to a person's physical body, gender concerns the way the person inhabiting that physical body feels, behaves, and is "read" by society.
- Individuals may communicate their internal sense of their gender (their gender identity) to those around them through the way they present their physical self (their gender expression) in the form of clothing, grooming or styling, and so on.
- When you are working with a patient whose assigned sex at birth and gender identity do not match, don't assume that the patient has had (or wants to have) surgery to bring their anatomy into alignment with their gender identity.
- Gender identity is distinct from sexual orientation.

- The only way to determine a person's sexual orientation is to ask—sexual orientation cannot be inferred from observed or even self-reported sexual behavior.
- To gather relevant clinical information about sex and gender, you need to ask patients two questions (ideally at the time of admission or intake): (1) What sex were you assigned at birth? and (2) What gender do you identify as now?
- Sexual health is as achievable and reasonable a goal for patients in palliative care and hospice care as pain relief. Sexual health should be part of the assessment and plan for every patient receiving palliative and hospice care.

DISCUSSION QUESTIONS

1. If a patient is assigned the female sex at birth, has a male gender identity and expression, self-identifies as male, and is attracted primarily to people who are biologically female and self-identify as female, what is this patient's sexual orientation? How did you come to this conclusion?

2. Imagine that you are working with a patient who was assigned a male sex at birth and has a female gender identity and presentation. The patient, Susan, is being admitted to a long-term care facility. As you arrange for Susan's admission what information, if any, should you provide to the facility regarding Susan's assigned sex at birth and her gender identity and expression? Should you request that Susan be assigned a female roommate or male roommate? Why?

3. Imagine that you have walked into a patient's room and found the patient masturbating. What do you do? Do you say anything? If so, what? What thoughts and feelings do you think you would experience in this situation?

4. Now imagine that *you* are the patient in that scenario. A health care professional has just walked into your room while you are masturbating. What do you do? Do you say

anything? If so, what? What thoughts and feelings do you think you would experience in this situation?

5. How many times in an average day do you think you "come out" — as straight, gay, lesbian, or bisexual — to people around you? Is this something you do deliberately or is it largely an unconscious act? Do you think it would be difficult to hide your sexual orientation for a day? For a week? For a month?

CHAPTER ACTIVITY

For the next week, hide your sexual orientation from everyone you come in contact with. To prepare for the possibility that a visitor may stop by your home or apartment, make sure to hide any photos, books, posters, or other items that might help visitors deduce your sexual orientation. During this week, you may not refer to a spouse or significant other using pronouns that would indicate what their gender is, and you may not hold hands, flirt, or otherwise demonstrate affection in public. Keep a journal throughout the week about your thoughts and feelings during this experience. How much energy did it take to hide who you are from other people? How has this experience changed your thoughts and feelings about the importance of LGBTQ-inclusive care?

CHAPTER 3

UNDERSTANDING ATTITUDES AND ACCESS TO CARE

CHAPTER OBJECTIVES

1. Explain how historical, political, institutional, and sociocultural factors may influence attitudes about palliative care and hospice among LGBTQ people.
2. Describe barriers faced by LGBTQ individuals and their families in accessing hospice and palliative care services.

Key Terms: access to care, barriers to care, employment discrimination, financial barriers to care, institutional barriers to care, perceptual barriers to care

CHAPTER SUMMARY

An important aspect of providing LGBTQ-inclusive care is understanding why some LGBTQ people may be reluctant either to seek care in the first place or to share with you that they are lesbian, gay, bisexual, transgender, gender nonconforming, queer, or questioning. Historically, disclosing one's status as an LGBTQ person has often come with a high price —and may still do so today. This chapter explains why, given the historical and contemporary contexts within which LGBTQ people live, it's not surprising that some LGBTQ patients and

Acquaviva, Kimberly
LGBTQ-Inclusive Hospice and Palliative Care
dx.doi.org/10.17312/harringtonparkpress/2017.03lgbtqihpc.003
© 2017 by Kimberly Acquaviva

families are reluctant to seek care. The chapter describes three kinds of barriers to palliative care and hospice care (perceptual, financial, and institutional) and offers a two-pronged approach to addressing barriers to care.

THE PAST AS PROLOGUE

William Shakespeare's words "what's past is prologue" ring especially true when it comes to understanding why some LGBTQ individuals may be fearful about accessing palliative or hospice care. When a person is diagnosed with a chronic or life-limiting illness, their past experiences with health care providers may shape their openness to receiving palliative care or hospice care. Because of the intersectionality of prejudice and social identity, LGBTQ persons may legitimately **fear** they will receive poor care or unfair treatment based on a combination of factors, including their race, ethnicity, sexual orientation, gender identity, gender expression, religion, and socioeconomic status. These fears may be based on firsthand experience, secondhand stories from family and friends, or thirdhand historical accounts.

Access to care, defined as "the timely use of personal health services to achieve the best health outcomes" (IOM 1993), is an issue of concern regarding the LGBTQ population. In a study of almost five thousand LGBTQ individuals, 56 percent of lesbian, gay, or bisexual respondents and 70 percent of gender nonconforming and transgender respondents reported having had at least one of the following experiences: "being refused needed care; health care professionals refusing to touch them or using excessive precautions; health care professionals using harsh or abusive language; being blamed for their health status; or health care professionals being physically rough or abusive" (Lambda Legal 2010). Among transgender and gender-nonconforming respondents, close to 21 percent reported that they had been "subjected to harsh or abusive language from a health care professional" (ibid.).

When issues of race, cultural tradition, and socioeconomic status intersect with or are layered on top of sexual orientation, gender identity, and gender expression, the effects of discrimination and poor-quality care are magnified: nearly 33 percent of low-income gender-nonconforming and transgender respondents in the Lambda Legal study said they had been refused care because of their gender identity (Lambda Legal 2010). More than 50 percent of lesbian, gay, and bisexual respondents and almost 86 percent of transgender respondents stated that "overall community fear or dislike of people like them is a barrier to care" (ibid.).

All patients you meet with bring with them their own complex set of experiences, beliefs, and fears, any or all of which may influence how they perceive and receive the care you extend to them. Knowing how to provide LGBTQ-inclusive care requires an understanding of the intersectionality of oppression and an awareness of how LGBTQ individuals have been treated in the United States over the past, say, seventy-five years. (While I could discuss a more extensive history of discrimination against LGBTQ persons in the United States, focusing on the past seventy-five years [1940–2016] will cover the lived experience of LGBTQ individuals age eighty and up, as well as provide a relatively recent history for younger LGBTQ individuals.

BEING LGBTQ COULD (AND STILL CAN) COST YOU YOUR JOB

At the beginning of the Cold War and the anticommunist McCarthy era in the United States, the federal government secretly investigated the lives of government employees in an attempt to ferret out those who were homosexual. The U.S. Senate issued a report to Congress in 1950 titled *Employment of Homosexuals and Other Sex Perverts in Government,* asserting that homosexuals constituted a security risk because "those who engage in overt acts of perversion lack the emotional stability of normal persons." In what became known as the "Lavender Scare," more than 4,300 gay men and lesbians

As a fifty-nine-year-old LGBT person, I grew up in an environment that was extremely homophobic. I was traumatized both within my family structure and within the community. LGBT seniors of my age were often exposed to various forms of psychological trauma, emotional trauma, and the mental trauma of isolation as well as not being able to be open about themselves. In addition, there are people such as myself who experienced quite severe physical trauma, assault, being stalked —actual life endangerment. As a cancer patient, [I found] the discrimination continued during the initial medical and surgical treatments. At the moment, though, I am also receiving palliative care, which to me is a godsend.

When I am talking about palliative care, I am talking about the whole gamut of psychiatry, social work, the total picture for all the psychosocial support that needs to be present for a cancer patient to successfully negotiate treatment. It is absolutely essential, and many people would fare so much better [in] cancer care and their symptoms would be managed much better if they were connected to palliative care.

—JAY KALLIO, TRANSGENDER ADVOCATE AND CANCER SURVIVOR

Author's note: Jay died on September 30, 2016, before this book went to press. Jay wanted to be listed as a "transgender advocate and cancer survivor," so I've honored his choice by listing him as such.

were discharged from the military and more than 500 civilians were fired from their jobs in the federal government (WGBH Educational Foundation 2011).

In 1953 the president of the United States, Dwight Eisenhower, issued Executive Order 10450, banning homosexuals, alcoholics, and "neurotics" from working for the government or its contractors. The ban was based on the perception that homosexuals, alcoholics, and neurotics posed a risk to national security (WGBH Educational Foundation 2011). On June 3, 1953, President Eisenhower said in his televised report to the American people regarding Executive Order 10450, "Employees could be a security risk and still not be disloyal or have any traitorous thoughts, but it may be that their personal habits are such that they might be subject to black-mail by people who seek to destroy the safety of our country" (Eisenhower 1953).

From 1950 to 1981 it was legal in every state in the United States to fire someone from their job because of their sexual orientation. During this period, in an attempt to pro-vide some city-level protections to LGBTQ people, some cities put in place antidiscrimination ordinances. In 1972 the mayor of New York City, for example, put in place antibias protec-tions for city employees fighting against **employment dis-crimination** based on sexual orientation (Torres n.d.). The first *state* to make it illegal to discriminate against someone on the basis of sexual orientation was Wisconsin, in 1982 (WGBH Educational Foundation 2011).

As of January 2016, it was still legal in the following twenty-eight states to deny a person employment — or to fire them from their current job — based solely on their sexual orientation or gender identity: Alabama, Alaska, Arizona, Arkansas, Florida, Georgia, Idaho, Indiana, Kansas, Kentucky, Louisiana, Michigan, Mississippi, Missouri, Montana, Nebraska, North Carolina, North Dakota, Ohio, Oklahoma, Pennsylvania, South Carolina, South Dakota, Tennessee, Texas, Virginia, West Virginia, and Wyoming (Movement Advancement Project 2016).

BEING LGBTQ COULD CAUSE YOU TO BE LABELED "MENTALLY ILL"

When the American Psychiatric Association's *Diagnostic and Statistical Manual of Mental Disorders* (*DSM*) was first pub-lished in 1952, it listed homosexuality as a form of sociopathy, and homosexuality continued to be classified as a mental illness for the next twenty years. The American Psychiatric Association (APA) finally removed homosexuality from its official list of mental illnesses in 1973 (WGBH Educational Foundation 2011).

The APA has made similar shifts in the way it classifies individuals whose assigned sex at birth does not align with their current self-identified gender. When the association added gender identity disorder to the *DSM* in 1980, the new diagnosis attached the stigmatizing label "disorder" to transgender individuals. In 2013, more than thirty years after it first attempted to put a label on the psychological state of transgender individuals, the APA issued a statement prior to the release of the fifth edition of the *DSM* (*DSM-5*), explaining that the term *gender identity disorder* was being replaced with *gender dysphoria*. In that statement, the APA said, "*DSM-5* aims to avoid stigma and ensure clinical care for individuals who see and feel themselves to be a different gender than their assigned gender. It replaces the diagnostic name 'gender identity disorder' with 'gender dysphoria,' as well as makes other important clarifications in the criteria. It is important to note that gender nonconformity is not in itself a mental disorder. The critical element of gender dysphoria is the presence of clinically significant distress associated with the condition" (APA 2013a).

The APA went on to explain why it had not removed the "condition" as a diagnosis altogether: "To get insurance coverage for the medical treatments, individuals need a diagnosis. The Sexual and Gender Identity Disorders Work Group was concerned that removing the condition as a psychiatric diagnosis—as some had suggested—would jeopardize access to care" (APA 2013a).

BEING LGBTQ COULD (AND STILL CAN) GET YOU EVICTED
In a national survey of 6,450 individuals who identified as transgender or gender nonconforming, 19 percent said they

had been homeless because of their gender identity, and 19 percent said they had been refused housing for the same reason (Grant et al. 2011). The U.S. Department of Housing and Urban Development (HUD) requires recipients of HUD funding to comply with laws at the state and local level that prohibit **housing discrimination** on the basis of sexual orientation and gender identity (HUD 2011). Yet as of January 2016 it was still legal in the following twenty-eight states to deny a person housing—or to evict them from their existing housing—based solely on their sexual orientation or gender identity: Alabama, Alaska, Arizona, Arkansas, Florida, Georgia, Idaho, Indiana, Kansas, Kentucky, Louisiana, Michigan, Mississippi, Missouri, Montana, Nebraska, North Carolina, North Dakota, Ohio, Oklahoma, Pennsylvania, South Carolina, South Dakota, Tennessee, Texas, Virginia, West Virginia, and Wyoming (Movement Advancement Project 2016).

BEING LGBTQ COULD (AND STILL CAN) GET YOU ARRESTED

Until 1962 sodomy was a crime in every state in the United States. That year, Illinois became the first state to decriminalize sodomy (WGBH Educational Foundation 2011), and in the 1970s **sodomy laws** were repealed in nineteen other states: California, Colorado, Connecticut, Delaware, Hawaii, Indiana, Iowa, Maine, Nebraska, New Jersey, New Mexico, North Dakota, Ohio, Oregon, South Dakota, Vermont, Washington, West Virginia, and Wyoming (ACLU n.d.).

The US Supreme Court ruled in 2003 that barring consensual sex between adults is unconstitutional. But in 2016— thirteen years after the Supreme Court ruling— consenting adults could still be arrested on charges of sodomy in twelve states: Alabama, Florida, Idaho, Kansas, Louisiana, Michigan, Mississippi, North Carolina, Oklahoma, South Carolina, Texas, and Utah. However, because states may not enforce unconstitutional laws, such cases have ended up being dropped (Coble 2015).

BEING LGBTQ COULD (AND STILL CAN) GET YOU ASSAULTED OR KILLED

In 1998 in Laramie, Wyoming, a twenty-one-year-old man named Matthew Shepard was tied to a split-rail fence, beaten, and left to die because he was gay (Human Rights Campaign n.d.). Twelve years after Matthew Shepard's murder, groundbreaking federal hate crimes legislation was enacted:

> The Matthew Shepard and James Byrd, Jr., Hate Crimes Prevention Act of 2009, 18 U.S.C. § 249, was enacted as Division E of the National Defense Authorization Act for Fiscal Year 2010. Section 249 of Title 18 provides funding and technical assistance to state, local, and tribal jurisdictions to help them to more effectively investigate and prosecute hate crimes. It also creates a new federal criminal law which criminalizes willfully causing bodily injury (or attempting to do so with fire, firearm, or other dangerous weapon) when: (1) the crime was committed because of the actual or perceived race, color, religion, national origin of any person or (2) the crime was committed because of the actual or perceived religion, national origin, gender, sexual orientation, gender identity, or disability of any person and the crime affected interstate or foreign commerce or occurred within federal special maritime and territorial jurisdiction. (DOJ 2009)

As of January 2016, six states still had no law against hate crimes: Arkansas, Georgia, Indiana, Michigan, South Carolina, and Wyoming. Of the states with hate crime laws, fourteen states — Alabama, Alaska, Idaho, Mississippi, Montana, North Carolina, North Dakota, Ohio, Oklahoma, Pennsylvania, South Dakota, Utah, Virginia, and West Virginia — did not outlaw hate crimes based on sexual orientation or gender identity (Movement Advancement Project 2016).

Sadly, LGBTQ people face threats to their physical safety even in states that have hate crime laws on their books. On June 12, 2016, the LGBTQ community in Orlando, Florida, was the target of the deadliest mass shooting by a sole gun-man in US history. The attack, which took place in Pulse, an LGBTQ nightclub, left forty-nine victims dead and more than fifty injured; many of the victims were both LGBTQ and Latino or Latina. As you read the list of the names and ages of those who were murdered in Orlando (City of Orlando 2016), reflect on how this attack and other hate crimes would be likely to affect LGBTQ individuals in your community, especially regarding how comfortable they feel about sharing who they are with people they have never met before:

Stanley Almodovar III, 23
Amanda Alvear, 25
Oscar A. Aracena-Montero, 26
Rodolfo Ayala-Ayala, 33
Antonio Davon Brown, 29
Darryl Roman Burt II, 29
Angel L. Candelario-Padro, 28
Juan Chevez-Martinez, 25
Luis Daniel Conde, 39
Cory James Connell, 21
Tevin Eugene Crosby, 25
Deonka Deidra Drayton, 32
Leroy Valentin Fernandez, 25
Simon Adrian Carrillo Fernandez, 31
Mercedez Marisol Flores, 26
Peter O. Gonzalez-Cruz, 22
Juan Ramon Guerrero, 22
Paul Terrell Henry, 41
Frank Hernandez, 27
Miguel Angel Honorato, 30
Javier Jorge-Reyes, 40
Jason Benjamin Josaphat, 19
Eddie Jamoldroy Justice, 30
Anthony Luis Laureanodisla, 25
Christopher Andrew Leinonen, 32

Alejandro Barrios Martinez, 21

Brenda Lee Marquez McCool, 49

Gilberto Ramon Silva Menendez, 25

Kimberly Morris, 37

Akyra Monet Murray, 18

Luis Omar Ocasio-Capo, 20

Geraldo A. Ortiz-Jimenez, 25

Eric Ivan Ortiz-Rivera, 36

Joel Rayon Paniagua, 32

Jean Carlos Mendez Perez, 35

Enrique L. Rios Jr., 25

Jean C. Nives Rodriguez, 27

Xavier Emmanuel Serrano Rosado, 35

Christopher Joseph Sanfeliz, 24

Yilmary Rodriguez Solivan, 24

Edward Sotomayor Jr., 34

Shane Evan Tomlinson, 33

Martin Benitez Torres, 33

Jonathan Antonio Camuy Vega, 24

Franky Jimmy Dejesus Velazquez, 50

Juan P. Rivera Velazquez, 37

Luis S. Vielma, 22

Luis Daniel Wilson-Leon, 37

Jerald Arthur Wright, 31

I have listed the victims' names because the phrase "forty-nine people died" doesn't come close to capturing the scope of the tragedy. Each life lost was a person — an individual whose death left an indelible mark on the LGBTQ community and whose name should not be forgotten. As you work with patients and families in the months and years to come, remember these victims and the effect their murders have had on the LGBTQ community. Not everyone will feel safe sharing who they are with you; patients and families should not have to "come out" to you in order to receive LGBTQ-inclusive care.

Given the long and ongoing history of discrimination against LGBTQ people in the United States, it is not surprising that LGBTQ individuals may be hesitant to seek health care of any sort, including palliative care or hospice care. For LGBTQ individuals, **barriers to care** fall into three general categories: (1) **perceptual barriers to care**, (2) **financial barriers to care**, and (3) **institutional barriers to care**. Understanding these barriers will be helpful as you work toward understanding the perspective of LGBTQ patients and families. Chapter 10 provides detailed information about ways that you and your employer or institution can ameliorate or eliminate these barriers in order to ensure greater inclusion of LGBTQ individuals.

PERCEPTUAL BARRIERS

For LGBTQ individuals with chronic or life-limiting illnesses, perceptual barriers to care may be twofold. Like their cisgender and heterosexual counterparts, LGBTQ individuals may have some of the same negative beliefs or fears about palliative care and hospice care. Common myths and misperceptions about palliative care include:

- If I receive palliative care, my pharmacy benefit will change and I won't be able to have chemotherapy or surgery.
- Palliative care is just another term for hospice care.
- If I receive palliative care, I'll have to change my primary care provider. (Paxton 2015).

Some common myths and misperceptions about hospice care include:

- Hospice is for people with cancer, not people with other illnesses or conditions.
- Hospice is a place—a physical facility sort of like a nursing home.

Sarah lives with two partners, an MtF* woman (Iris) who she was previously married to before Iris transitioned, and Damian, a cis man. Sarah described a period of time recently when she was [feeling] very poorly and [was] in [the] hospital. When she came home she convalesced in a room set up especially for her. She went on to explain: "It was difficult to explain to anybody coming in why this was a change. They would come in, they would see me in that single bed in that single room, and they would see Damian and Iris, and even if they accepted that we are three, they would see they had the main bedroom, and they wouldn't realize or understand that actually normally I would have been in there too, and I would be missing it."

— KATHRYN ALMACK, PHD

*MtF is used as shorthand for "male-to-female," indicating that the individual was assigned the male sex at birth but identifies as female. Passage is from *The Last Outing: Exploring End of Life Experiences and Care Needs in the Lives of Older LGBT People* (Almack et al. 2014).

- If I'm admitted to hospice, it means I have given up hope.
- Hospice care costs a lot of money (Naierman and Turner 2012).

LGBTQ individuals may also have fears or concerns specific to their gender identity, gender expression, or sexual orientation, in addition to the common misperceptions about hospice and palliative care that many people share. Special concerns about hospice and palliative care for LGBTQ individuals may include:

- I will be refused care because of my gender identity, gender expression, or sexual orientation.

- I will have to spend my limited time and energy educating my health care providers.
- I'll be treated like a pariah or a freak.
- I will have to hide evidence of my gender identity or sexual orientation (e.g., photos, books) in my home so that my health care providers won't figure out I'm LGBTQ.
- I'll run the risk of being "outed" to my family members.
- I will be treated politely enough, but the care I receive will somehow be less than what others receive.

FINANCIAL BARRIERS

For individuals who have private insurance, Medicare, or Medicaid, palliative care and hospice care are covered either in part or in total. However, because of the complexity of health care costs, copays, and insurance coverage, LGBTQ individuals (like their cisgender and heterosexual counterparts) may be unsure how much their out-of-pocket cost would be for palliative care or hospice care. Transgender patients receiving hormone therapy may worry that a hospice admission would cause them to lose pharmacy coverage for their hormones. They may also fear that the hospice wouldn't understand that it's essential that patients remain on hormones for the rest of their life if that's their preference. For LGBTQ individuals who do not have health care insurance, financial concerns will be even more pressing.

INSTITUTIONAL BARRIERS

Hospice and palliative care programs may unintentionally erect barriers that prevent LGBTQ individuals from accessing their services. Such institutional barriers can include discriminatory admission and employment policies; noninclusive marketing and outreach materials; and inadequate orientation and training for health care providers, staff, and volunteers. If your institution's nondiscrimination statement does not include gender identity, gender expression, and sexual orientation, you will have a difficult time convincing LGBTQ

Back [in the 1990s], we identified the "primary caregiver" on a written fact sheet, by name and relationship to the patient. Most of the time, same-sex partners were listed as "friend" under "relationship to patient." When you think about issues like anticipatory grief and role/relationship changes due to illness, "friend" is not a word that adequately conveys what partners were likely going through. I had several patients tell me the nature of their relationship and ask me not to share [it] with other team members, I assume for fear it would somehow affect their care. I always believed they knew best, and I never shared what I was asked to keep in confidence.

—KATHLEEN TAYLOR, MA, LMHC

individuals to enter your program for palliative or hospice care.

Addressing institutional barriers to care requires a two-pronged approach: outward facing and inward looking. The outward-facing approach to addressing these barriers involves creating outreach and educational materials (e.g., a website, brochures) that specifically address LGBTQ individuals' myths, misperceptions, and concerns about hospice and palliative care. The inward-looking aspect of addressing institutional barriers to care is even more important. It requires teaching all caregivers, staff, and volunteers how to provide inclusive care to LGBTQ individuals and their families — "to promote comfort and acceptance, identify and diminish bias[,] . . . minimize heterosexual assumptions within assessment and care, and thus strengthen open communication" (Harding, Epiphaniou, and Chidgey-Clark 2012). To illustrate this, imagine the care your institution provides is a box of pasta. Changing how people with celiac disease perceive and experience your company's pasta goes beyond simply slapping a "gluten- free" label on the box. Unless you change how you make the pasta, your company's product will continue to be harmful to people who consume it.

KEY POINTS TO REMEMBER

- All patients bring their own complex sets of experiences, beliefs, and fears to their interactions with you, any or all of which may influence the way in which they perceive and receive the care you extend to them.
- Understanding how to provide LGBT-inclusive care requires an understanding of the intersectionality of oppression and an awareness of the ways in which LGBTQ individuals have been treated in the United States over the past seventy-five years.
- For LGBTQ individuals, barriers to palliative care and hospice care fall into three general categories: (1) perceptual barriers, (2) financial barriers, and (3) institutional barriers.
- Addressing barriers to care requires a two-pronged approach on the part of your hospice or palliative care program: outward facing and inward looking.
- **Outward facing:** Create outreach and educational materials that address LGBTQ individuals' myths, misperceptions, and concerns about hospice and palliative care.
- **Inward looking:** Teach all care providers, staff, and volunteers how to provide inclusive care to LGBTQ patients and families.

DISCUSSION QUESTIONS

1. Imagine that you are working with Bob, an eighty-five-year-old man who lives with Doug, his "best friend" of sixty years. Bob and Doug have been very reluctant to access home health care services to help Bob with showering, a task he says has become too difficult for him and Doug to manage. What are some of the historical, political, institutional, and sociocultural factors that may have influenced Bob and Doug's attitude toward seeking

and receiving care? Would Bob need to "come out" to the interdisciplinary/interprofessional team in order to receive optimal care? Why or why not?

2. What are some of the barriers faced by LGBTQ individuals and their families in accessing hospice and palliative care services? What are some reasons LGBTQ individuals might be hesitant to seek services from a palliative care or hospice program in your community?

3. If given a choice, would you prefer to be assigned a cis-gender heterosexual ("straight") patient or a transgender heterosexual patient? What if the choice were between being assigned a cisgender gay patient or a cisgender straight patient? Why? Do you think your preferences are similar to those of your colleagues in the field or different?

4. Perceptual barriers to care for LGBTQ patients include general misperceptions and concerns about palliative care and hospice care as well as concerns specific to their status as LGBTQ individuals. Given the subjectivity of "perception," how can palliative care and hospice programs address perceptual barriers to care?

5. Imagine that you are working in a palliative care or hospice program that has decided to address barriers to care for LGBTQ people. Describe how you might address institutional barriers to care using both outward-facing and inward-looking strategies. Which set of strategies would you recommend tackling first: outward facing or inward looking? Why?

CHAPTER ACTIVITY

In the state where you live, what laws, if any, protect LGBTQ individuals from discrimination? How do you think these laws (or their absence) affect the degree to which LGBTQ individuals in your community feel safe and comfortable seeking hospice or palliative care? Visit http://www.lambdalegal.org/in-your-state to find information about your state.

CHAPTER 4

THE HISTORY AND PHYSICAL EXAMINATION

CHAPTER OBJECTIVES

1. Identify the five dimensions of a comprehensive history for palliative care and hospice patients, including relevant information about the patient's anatomy, birth sex, gender identity, sexual orientation, sexual behavior, and sexual health.

2. Distinguish between questions that are relevant and necessary to your care of the patient and questions that may stem primarily from your personal curiosity about a patient's life or body.

3. Identify the necessary and appropriate elements of the physical examination for palliative care and hospice patients.

4. Describe how to assess and support "diverse cultural values and customs with regard to information sharing, decision making, expression and treatment of physical and emotional distress, and preferences for sites of care and death" (AAHPM 2009).

Key Terms: chosen family, comprehensive history, family of choice, family of origin, FICA Spiritual History Tool, Five-Dimension Assessment Model, gender-affirmation surgery, Patient and Family Outcomes-Focused Inquiry for Developing Goals for Care, Patient and Family Outcomes-Focused Inquiry for Interdisciplinary Teams, patient's goals of care, prognosis, psychosocial history, quality of life, rapport, spiritual/ existential history

Acquaviva, Kimberly
LGBTQ-Inclusive Hospice and Palliative Care
dx.doi.org/10.17312/harringtonparkpress/2017.03lgbtqihpc.004
© 2017 by Kimberly Acquaviva

To elicit a complete and accurate history from a patient, palliative care and hospice professionals need to establish rapport and communicate a genuine openness to hearing the patient's answers to their questions. This chapter describes a new LGBTQ-inclusive approach to taking a comprehensive history that places the primary emphasis on the patient as person. Pathophysiology, pharmacology, and differential diagnoses are beyond the scope of *LGBTQ-Inclusive Hospice and Palliative Care;* this chapter provides information to supplement readers' existing clinical expertise and knowledge.

AN EVIDENCE-BASED APPROACH TO TAKING A COMPREHENSIVE HISTORY

If you have not already done so, take a close look at the National Quality Forum's *National Voluntary Consensus Standards: Palliative and End-of-Life Care — A Consensus Report* (2012). Hospice and palliative care providers are encouraged to use these evidence-based measures to collect and report data publicly on the care delivered. The care you deliver to patients and families should support your program's efforts to deliver care that meets the National Quality Forum's endorsed measures for palliative care and end-of-life care, summarized in table 4.1.

In its *Clinical Practice Guidelines for Quality Palliative Care,* the National Consensus Project for Quality Palliative Care (2013) provides direction regarding elements of the history-taking process according to criteria delineated under six domains:

- Domain 1: Structure and Processes of Care
- Domain 2: Physical Aspects of Care
- Domain 3: Psychological and Psychiatric Aspects of Care
- Domain 4: Social Aspects of Care
- Domain 5: Spiritual, Religious, and Existential Aspects of Care
- Domain 6: Cultural Aspects of Care

Domain	National Quality Forum–endorsed measures
Pain management	Hospice and palliative care—pain screening
	Hospice and palliative care—pain assessment
	Patients treated with an opioid who are given a bowel regimen
	Patients with advanced cancer assessed for pain at outpatient visits
Dyspnea management	Hospice and palliative care—dyspnea screening
	Hospice and palliative care—dyspnea treatment
Care preference	Patients admitted to ICU who have care preferences documented
	Hospice and palliative care—treatment preferences
	Percentage of hospice patients with documentation in the clinical record of a discussion of spiritual/religious concerns, or documentation that the patient/caregiver did not want to discuss
Quality of care at the end of life	Comfortable dying
	Hospitalized patients who die an expected death with an Implantable Cardioverter Defribillator (ICD) that has been deactivated
	Family evaluation of hospice care
	CARE—Consumer Assessments and Reports of End of Life
	Bereaved-family survey

Source: National Quality Forum 2012. Table text © 2012 The National Quality Forum.
Reprinted with permission.

To elicit a complete and accurate history, providers need to establish a **rapport** with each patient and communicate a genuine openness to hearing the patient's answers to their questions. A **comprehensive history** should never be viewed as a checklist or form you have to fill out. With the advent of electronic health records and computer-based charting, the process of taking and documenting a patient's history has, in many care settings, become less intimate and more robotic. A health care provider sits facing a computer, asking their patient a series of questions while clicking and scrolling through a checklist and drop-down menus. What health care providers gain in efficiency they lose in effectiveness, owing to the loss of connection.

In palliative care and hospice care, physicians, APRNs, and RNs can elicit the most complete and accurate history by using the old-school tools of the caring professions: **eye contact**, genuine **listening**, and a pencil and paper. By sitting across from a patient, looking the person in the eye, and giving the individual your full attention, you will facilitate the patient's willingness to open up to you and provide an accurate history.

You may be reading this and thinking to yourself, "There's no time for doing it the way you're suggesting and then charting it in the electronic health record after I leave the visit with the patient. If I don't type it into the electronic record while I'm meeting with the patient, I won't have time to get everything done." I'm a huge fan of technology as a time-saver, but when it comes to taking a comprehensive history from a

PROVIDER PERSPECTIVE

What not to do: assum[e] you know who the patient/client is because he/she is LGBT. It's not meant to be cruel—I know when providers are doing this they're trying to create a trusting bond. The problem is that they're doing it without waiting to find out who the patient/client is. Experiences I've had/observed: providers assuming a gay man identifies with female pronouns/references, providers trying to figure out who in a gay relationship is the "man" and who is the "woman," and "fag hag" providers who love gay men and assume they must be like her gay best friend.

—RICHARD GOLLANCE, LCSW, MSG

patient, I am firmly in the Luddite camp. By eliciting a complete and accurate history—and building the rapport needed to do so—you will save time in the long run. An assessment should be more of a conversation than an interrogation, so make sure your questions flow naturally and organically.

COORDINATING AND FACILITATING THE FIRST FAMILY MEETING

As a member of the interdisciplinary/interprofessional team, you are likely to play a role in coordinating and facilitating family meetings. What that role looks like will vary, depending on your discipline, the size of the program where you work, and the particular needs of each patient and family. What the interdisciplinary/interprofessional team looks like will vary as well. If you work in a hospital-based palliative care program, for example, you may be part of a palliative care consultation team. Because Medicare and Medicaid require that the initial assessment of a hospice patient be completed by a registered nurse, an RN on the interdisciplinary/interprofessional team is likely to be the person coordinating the first family meeting for a hospice patient. Within palliative care, a physician or advanced practice RN will likely convene the first family meeting.

You may not think of the first time you meet with a patient as a "family meeting." After all, your focus during the first meeting is typically on taking a comprehensive history, conducting a **physical examination**, and identifying the patient's goals for care. But when you treat your first meeting with a patient as a family meeting, you will clearly establish from the outset your respect for and recognition of the patient and family as the unit of care. If the patient and family truly *are* the unit of care, every interaction with a patient should take this into account. Thus, the way you coordinate and facilitate the first meeting sets the tone for all your future interactions with the patient and family. So what is a "family"? Many people have two kinds of families: the family they were born or adopted into (sometimes called their **family of origin**) and the group of close friends they have chosen to surround themselves with, sometimes called their **chosen family**, their **family of choice**, or, among some LGBTQ people, their "lavender family" (Lawton, White, and Fromme 2014; Neville and Henrickson 2009; Rawlings 2012). When arranging the first meeting, always ask patients whom they consider to be their family and whom they would like to have present at the meeting. The way you ask this question will communicate the degree to which you're open to a variety of familial configurations, so be intentional in your choice of language. For example, instead of asking a female patient, "Would you like to bring your husband or boyfriend?" ask, "Whom do you consider to be your family? Who are the people in your life who are sources of emotional support for you?" Follow up by mentioning that many patients find it helpful to invite one or more people to participate in their meeting with the provider, then ask if that's something they might be open to. By suggesting that many patients find this helpful *before* you ask the patient if they want to bring someone to the meeting, you normalize the idea of bringing a support person. After a patient suggests one or more people they'd like to invite to the meeting, ask, "Is there anyone else you'd like to have there with you?" Some patients will have multiple family members and friends they would like to bring with them. This can present logistical challenges to you as a provider in terms of scheduling the meeting, but the effort you expend to ensure that the family meeting includes all the key players is worthwhile. Mention that some patients prefer to have the provider take their history and perform the physical exam with their family member(s) in the room, and some patients prefer that their family member(s) be invited into the room after the provider finishes taking their history and performing the physical exam. Then ask patients if they would like the people they named to be in the room for the physical exam and history, or only for the care planning discussion afterward.

It was incredibly validating when the nurse who was visiting my dad pointed to my partner and me and the dogs and said, "This is your family. You are surrounded by a beautiful family. What better way to be than that?"

—NICK KRAYGER, MSW

Once patients have identified the people they would like to have present at the family meeting, ask whether any of the individuals have mobility, hearing, or visual impairments that you should be aware of, in order to ensure their access to and full participation in the family meeting. In addition, ask whether any of the individuals will need an interpreter present. When you ask these questions, you communicate to patients that you see the involvement of their identified "family" as being vitally important to the care you provide. Enlist the help of the social worker or counselor on your interdisciplinary/interprofessional team to make the necessary arrangements for accommodating the needs of the family.

At your first meeting with the patient and family, check in with the patient again to see who they would like to have in the room during the physical exam and/or history, if anyone. If the patient has one or more family members who will be waiting outside the room until the history and physical are complete, offer them a quiet place to sit.

If one or more of the family members will be in the room with the patient, seat the patient and family member(s) in chairs at the same level as your chair or stool. Direct your questions to the patient but warmly acknowledge the presence of the family member(s), taking your cues from the patient as to how involved the family member(s) should be in the back-and-forth regarding the patient's history. If you notice the patient appearing agitated or impatient each time a family

My dad moved in with me over the Christmas holiday in 2012. I noticed his coloring was bad, his health ailing, and over the next two years he went from fully independent to mostly dependent for ADLs [activities of daily living], three-day-a-week dialysis treatment, and transport to all medical procedures and appointments. My father really fell ill in the fall of 2014, and I had to take leave from work. Over those two years, my dad was in and out of the hospital twenty-some times. We discussed his ailing health and he said he wanted to die at home, with me, surrounded by our wiener dogs. He explained what he wanted from his hospice experience, when the time came, and that he wanted to be at home with the dogs.

My dad decided on a Monday that he was stopping dialysis. He had already missed his regular Friday treatment. The doctor called me very matter-of-factly and said, "You realize it will be no more than seven to ten days." That hit like a ton of bricks. I knew that, but to have a doctor state it set it in stone: He [would] die within a week. There was no turning back.

My estranged lover had been gone about six months, and when I told him my dad was receiving hospice care and I was alone, he showed up with his dog and a suitcase and said he was there for the duration. He helped me every day through and past the end. My dad died a beautiful peaceful death. He had Chinese food for dinner. Took a sip of Angry Orchard beer, got last rites from our family priest, and then said to my lover and me, "Well, fellows, it looks like it's my time to go." He [lay] down in his bed. All five of our dogs climbed to their respective spots around him. I rubbed his head. My niece held his hand. We listened to *The Snowman* soundtrack play and turned the fire up high, with the windows wide open.

> My lover burned sage, and my dad peacefully left his body and this life within an hour—in his bed, with the ones he loved, surrounded by the dogs. That was his final wish. And it was perfect.
>
> —NICK KRAYGER, MSW

member answers a question, you might subtly turn your body more toward the patient (and away from the family member) and start your next question with the patient's name. For example, "Mary, you mentioned that you had surgery last year. Tell me a bit more about that."

DEVELOPMENT OF A NEW MODEL FOR ASSESSMENT

A comprehensive history generally contains the following:

- Assessment of the patient's **quality of life**
- Information about the patient's **advance directives** (living will, durable power of attorney for health care, health care proxy or surrogate)
- The patient's **goals of care**
- History of the patient's illness and physical **symptoms**
- The patient's understanding of the illness and **prognosis**
- **Psychosocial history** (including mental health diagnoses and previous treatment) and **spiritual/existential history**
- The patient's birth sex and gender identity
- Sexual orientation and sexual behavior
- Surgical history
- Assessment of patient's activities of daily living (ADLs)
- Depression screening
- List of pharmacologic, nonpharmacologic, and complementary/alternative therapies
- List of allergies and drug interactions
- Information regarding substance abuse or dependency

Because of the large amount of information you need to gather when taking a comprehensive history, it is helpful to have an organizing framework to follow. Unfortunately, the only place I have found even the roughest beginnings of a clear map of questions clinicians should ask patients and families is Knight and von Gunten's *Module 3: Whole-Patient Assessment: Nine Dimensions* (2004), which is a core component of *The Education in Palliative and End-of-Life Care (EPEC) Curriculum* (Emanuel et al. 1999–2011).

Each discipline has core texts that are foundational to that particular field and that delineate key questions to ask in certain areas, but I have never seen anything in print that covers the waterfront in a unified way that all the disciplines can work with. The National Consensus Project for Quality Palliative Care's *Clinical Practice Guidelines for Quality Palliative Care* (2013) comes closest to a multidisciplinary approach in its identification of "eight important domains in the creation and maintenance of quality palliative care[:] Structure and Processes, Physical Aspects of Care, Psychosocial and Psychiatric Aspects of Care, Social Aspects of Care, Spiritual, Religious, and Existential Aspects of Care, Cultural Aspects of Care, Care of the Patient at the End of Life, and Ethical and Legal Aspects of Care." The National Consensus Project (NCP) succeeds in providing "guidelines that delineate optimal practice . . . [and that] rest on the principles of assessment, information sharing, decision-making, care planning, and care delivery" (National Consensus Project for Quality Palliative Care 2013). Without a doubt, the NCP guidelines are a triumph in the arena of evidence-based practice. Where they fall short, however, is in explaining *how* to ask questions to meet the guidelines for quality palliative care—and how to ask them in an inclusive way.

It's hard for me to imagine someone reading the NCP guidelines and thinking, "No, I don't want to deliver quality palliative care." Where a clinician's good intentions fail to translate to behavior change is in the execution of those intentions.

Thus, one of my goals in writing this book and developing a new assessment model was to give clinicians a crystal-clear road map to asking questions and delivering care in an LGBTQ-inclusive manner. By design, this book isn't a dense read, nor is it a replacement for seminal works like the NCP guidelines or the Oxford Textbooks (see Altilio and Otis-Green 2011; Cherny et al. 2015; Ferrell, Coyle, and Paice 2015a). Instead, I am trying to teach clinicians about the language of inclusion in a practical way. As a starting point in developing an assessment model to accomplish this goal, I looked at Knight and von Gunten's *Whole-Patient Assessment: Nine Dimensions* (2004) and the framework it provides for palliative care and hospice care providers. The nine dimensions in their assessment are:

1. Illness/Treatment Summary
2. Physical
3. Psychological
4. Decision-Making
5. Communication and Information Sharing
6. Social
7. Spiritual/Existential
8. Practical
9. Anticipatory Planning for Death

A potential limitation of Knight and von Gunten's nine-dimension framework is the way in which it starts with the primary illness rather than with the patient as a human being. Although their framework is a nominal rather than ordinal listing of dimensions, the order in which the dimensions are listed could be interpreted as having some significance, even if none was intended. This approach runs the risk of medicalizing rather than humanizing the provider-patient interaction, sending the message to the patient that the provider's focus is on the illness, not on the person.

Given the limitations and gaps in the extant assessment models, I realized that a new, inclusive, patient-centered model was needed—a new assessment tool that I call the **Five-Dimension Assessment Model**. Based on a synthesis of the extant literature on patient and family assessment for palliative and hospice care, the Five-Dimension Assessment Model is designed to serve as a practical framework for a comprehensive patient history in palliative care and hospice care.

Knight and von Gunten's framework is focused more on the illness than on the patient. To address this problem, I added a dimension called "Patient as Person" at the beginning and end of the new framework and collapsed Knight and von Gunten's psychological, social, spiritual/existential, and communication and information sharing dimensions into this new dimension. Because the members of the interdisciplinary/interprofessional team share responsibility for supporting the patient's and family's plan of care in all domains, including the psychosocial and spiritual, I made a purposeful shift away from creating psychosocial and spiritual "silos"—stand-alone domains for psychosocial and spiritual care—in the new model. Finally, I incorporated elements of Knight and von Gunten's practical dimension into the other dimensions and changed the name of Knight and von Gunten's physical dimension to "Functional Activities and Symptoms," to remind providers of the focus of this aspect of the history-taking process.

In formulating the spiritual aspects of the Five-Dimension Assessment Model, I made use of Christina Puchalski's **FICA Spiritual History Tool** ©, a widely used model for assessing and addressing spiritual issues with patients (Puchalski 1996). While a variety of tools can be used for taking a spiritual history, I like the FICA Spiritual History Tool because it can be used by palliative care and hospice physicians, APRNs, RNs, social workers, counselors, and chaplains alike.

To foster inclusive care, the Five-Dimension Assessment Model incorporates questions about birth sex, gender identity, sexual orientation, sexual behavior, and sexual health in the assessment process and places the primary focus on the "patient as person." The five dimensions are:

- Dimension 1A: Patient as Person, Part 1
- Dimension 2: Illness/Treatment Summary
- Dimension 3: Functional Activities and Symptoms
- Dimension 4: Decision Making
- Dimension 5: Anticipatory Planning for Death
- Dimension 1B: Patient as Person, Part 2

The model is not intended as a research framework. Instead, I drew from the best of the evidence to develop a practical approach to providing inclusive care. To make the framework as useful as possible, I include assessment questions that clinicians can use in each dimension of the framework.

When someone is diagnosed with a chronic or life-limiting illness, their life changes in countless ways. Their diagnosis is likely to force them to make adjustments to their daily routine, priorities, long-term goals, and how they choose to spend their limited time and energy. **Fatigue**—both physical and emotional—can also take its toll on a patient with a chronic or life-limiting illness. These changes can affect a patient's desire for intimacy with a partner or spouse. One of the gaps I observed in Knight and von Gunten's framework was the absence of a sexual health assessment, and I have incorporated sexual health questions into Dimension 2 of the Five-Dimension Assessment Model. As the *Oxford Textbook of Palliative Nursing* notes, sexuality is an important component of the social aspects of palliative care (Ferrell, Coyle, and Paice 2015a).

USING THE FIVE-DIMENSION ASSESSMENT MODEL

When you first meet a patient, there is a narrow window of opportunity in which you can communicate your commitment to honoring the patient's values, customs, and preferences. Patients—particularly those who have had negative experiences with health care providers in the past—have an exquisitely fine-tuned radar for detecting health care providers who are closed-minded or focused on their own agenda. To address this, I have incorporated into the Five-Dimension Assessment Model questions about values, customs, and preferences (Golley 2012). Also, before you begin the assessment conversation outlined here, preface it by telling the patient how you plan to proceed and indicating that the patient will be in control of the process. You might say, for example, "I'm going to ask you a series of questions that I ask all the patients I work with. If you don't feel comfortable answering a particular question, feel free to let me know and we can skip it." (*Note:* The following is based on the assumption that the questions "What sex were you assigned at birth?" and "What gender do you identify as now?" were asked at the time of intake and the answers are documented in the patient's chart.)

DIMENSION 1A: PATIENT AS PERSON, PART 1

- What name would you like me to call you?
- What gender pronouns do you go by (e.g., he/him, she/her, them/their, ze/zir)?
- What word or words would you use to describe your sexual orientation?
- How would you describe your current quality of life?
- I'd like to learn more about your family. Many patients have two kinds of families: the family they were born or adopted into (sometimes called their family of origin) and the support group of close friends they have chosen to surround themselves with (what some people call their chosen family, family of choice, or lavender family).
- Who are the people you consider to be part of your family of origin? *For each person named, ask:*
  - How would you describe your relationship with _____?
  - Is your relationship with _____ generally a source of support or a source of stress?
  - Many people have unresolved differences or conflicts

that they want to resolve before they die. What, if any, unresolved differences do you have with _____?

- What role, if any, do you hope _____ will play in your care?

- Under the HIPAA Privacy Rule (45 CFR 164.510b), I can generally share information directly relevant to your care with your family and friends only if I have your permission to do so. What information, if any, would you like me to share with _____ regarding your illness, condition, or care?

- What information, if any, would you *not* want me to share with _____ regarding your illness, condition, or care?

- Who are the people you consider to be your family of choice? *For each person named, ask:*

  - How would you describe your relationship with _____?

  - Is your relationship with _____ generally a source of support or a source of stress?

  - Many people have unresolved differences or conflicts that they want to resolve before they die. What, if any, unresolved differences do you have with _____?

  - What role, if any, do you hope _____ will play in your care?

  - Under the HIPAA Privacy Rule (45 CFR 164.510b), I can generally share information directly relevant to your care with your family and friends only if I have your permission to do so. What information, if any, would you like me to share with _____ regarding your illness, condition, or care?

  - What information, if any, would you *not* want me to share with _____ regarding your illness, condition, or care?

- I'd like to learn about your connections and supports in your community. What groups or organizations do you belong to that are important to you?

- What role do these groups play in your life?
- What involvement, if any, have these groups or communities had in meeting your needs for care or support in the past?
- What involvement would you like them to have in the future?
- I'd like to learn about the things that give your life meaning or give you strength:
  - "Do you have spiritual or religious beliefs that help you cope with stress/difficult times? What gives your life meaning?" (Puchalski 1996).
  - "What importance does your spirituality have in your life? Has your spirituality influenced how you take care of yourself, your health? Does your spirituality influence you in your healthcare decision making (e.g. advance directives, treatment etc.)?" (Puchalski 1996).
  - "Are you part of a spiritual community? Communities such as churches, temples, and mosques, or a group of like-minded friends, family, or yoga, can serve as strong support systems for some patients. . . . Is this of support to you, and how? Is there a group of people you really love or who are important to you?" (Puchalski 1996).
  - "How would you like me, your healthcare provider, to address these issues in your healthcare?" (Puchalski 1996).
- I'd like to learn more about your informal social activities and hobbies. When you have free time, what are the kinds of things you like to do?
  - What role do these activities and/or hobbies play in your life?
  - What involvement would you like to have with these activities and/or hobbies in the future?
- I'd like to learn more about household supports and stressors. Many times, patients find themselves experiencing difficulty as a result of their chronic or life-limiting illness.

F — Faith/belief: Do you have spiritual or religious beliefs that help you cope with stress/difficult times? What gives your life meaning?

I — Importance: What importance does your spirituality have in your life? Has your spirituality influenced how you take care of yourself, your health? Does your spirituality influence you in your healthcare decision making (e.g., advance directives, treatment, etc.)?

C — Community: Are you part of a spiritual community? Communities such as churches, temples, and mosques, or a group of like-minded friends, family, or yoga, can serve as strong support systems for some patients. . . . Is this of support to you, and how? Is there a group of people you really love or who are important to you?

A — Address in care: How would you like me, your healthcare provider, to address these issues in your healthcare?

From Puchalski 1996. FICA © Christina Puchalski, MD; reprinted with permission. See also Puchalski 2014.

- Whom do you consider to be your primary caregiver?
- Who else is available to help you with your everyday needs?
- How are you managing financially in light of the illness you are currently facing?
- Who is in charge of your banking and paying your bills?
- How has your illness affected your ability to meet your other financial obligations, such as rent, mortgage, utility bills, and so on?
- Who does the grocery shopping and cooking in your house?

- Are there ever weeks when you are unable to afford enough groceries to meet your basic needs?
- Are there ever weeks when you're unable to afford your medications?
- How do you get to and from appointments?

DIMENSION 2: ILLNESS/TREATMENT SUMMARY

- What is the primary illness that brought you to [palliative care/hospice care]?
- How has that illness affected your life?
- What treatments, if any, have you received for that illness?
- How did those treatments affect your life?
- What is your understanding of your prognosis?
- How would you like us to share medical information with you? Would you prefer general "bullet points" or more detailed information? How would you like to receive this information: alone or with someone else—family, friends, etc.? Or would you rather not receive the information yourself and instead appoint someone else to receive it?
- What other illnesses or conditions do you have? *For each illness, ask:*
  - How has that illness affected your life?
  - What treatments, if any, did you receive for that illness?
  - How did those treatments affect your life?
- What prescription medications are you currently taking? *For each prescription medication, ask:*
  - Frequency?
  - Dose?
  - Reason prescribed?
  - Any adverse effects?
- What over-the-counter medications are you currently taking? *For each over-the-counter medication, ask:*
  - Frequency?

- Dose?
- Reason taking?
- Any adverse effects?
- What vitamins, supplements, and/or complementary/ alternative therapies are you currently taking? *For each vitamin, supplement, and/or complementary/alternative therapies, ask:*
  - Frequency?
  - Dose?
  - Reason taking?
  - Any adverse effects?
- What other drugs or hormones (either prescribed or obtained another way) are you currently taking? *For each additional drug and/or hormone, ask:*
  - Frequency?
  - Dose?
  - Reason taking?
  - Any adverse effects?
- Do you have any worries or concerns about your past or current substance use as it relates to your current care?
- Do you have any allergies or adverse reactions to any medications?
- Have you had any surgeries other than the ones you have already mentioned to me?
  - What was the reason for that surgery?
  - When did you have the surgery?
  - Were there any complications or problems after the surgery?
- One area of people's lives that rarely gets the attention needed from health care providers is sexuality. Some patients have never been asked questions like these before, so I want to let you know why I'm asking them. No matter a person's age or physical abilities or health conditions, sex and intimacy may be important aspects of that person's life. As a health care provider, I want to do whatever I can to ensure that this part of your life remains as

fulfilling as possible, to the extent that this is something that's important to you. May I ask you a few questions about this?

- What questions or concerns do you have about sex and intimacy in your life?
- Is sex with a partner, or other forms of sexual expression—whether partnered or not—important to you?
- Do you have any physical or health concerns regarding the act of masturbation (self-love) and/or sex with a partner or partners, such as pain, bleeding, difficulty reaching orgasm?
- What are some goals to optimize sexual function for you?

DIMENSION 3: FUNCTIONAL ACTIVITIES AND SYMPTOMS

Functional activities are often referred to as activities of daily living (ADLs) and instrumental activities of daily living (IADLs).

- What kind of help do you currently need with bathing? For example:
  - Do you need help getting undressed?
  - Do you need help getting in and out of the tub or shower?
  - Do you need help washing yourself?
- What kind of help do you currently need with dressing yourself? For example:
  - Do you need help getting your clothes out of your closet?
  - Do you need help buttoning shirts and pants?
  - Do you need help pulling shirts and sweaters over your head?
  - Do you need help bending down to put on your socks and shoes?
- What kind of help do you currently need with feeding yourself? For example:
  - Do you need help preparing your meals?
  - Do you need help carrying your meal to the table?

- Do you need help cutting your food with a knife?
- Do you need help using a spoon or fork?

- What kind of help do you currently need with changing positions or transferring your body from one location to another? For example:
  - Do you need help sitting up?
  - Do you need help getting out of bed?
  - Do you need help moving from your bed to a chair?
  - Do you need help moving from a chair to the bathroom?
  - Do you need help moving onto or off of the toilet?
  - Do you need help getting into or out of a car?
- What kind of help do you currently need managing bladder or bowel continence (aka urinating and having bowel movements)? For example:
  - Do you sometimes have accidents in which you don't make it to the bathroom in time?
  - Do these accidents happen frequently enough that you need to wear incontinence pads or adult diapers?
  - Are you able to wipe yourself?
- What kind of help do you currently need getting to the bathroom? For example:
  - Are you able to get to the bathroom without assistance?
  - Do you use a urinal, bedpan, or bedside commode at night because of difficulties making it to the bathroom in time?
- *When assessing each symptom—anxiety, breathlessness, confusion, constipation, depression, insomnia, nausea/vomiting, pain, weakness/fatigue, weight loss—ask:*
  - Have you experienced any _____ in the past week?
  - Are you currently experiencing any _____?
  - On a scale of 0 to 10, with 0 being no _____ and 10 being the worst _____ you can imagine, how would you rate your current _____?
  - How has your _____ interfered with your daily activities? With your sleeping? With your walking?

Consider using a valid, reliable assessment instrument like the Edmonton Symptom Assessment System (Bruera et al. 1991) or the Memorial Symptom Assessment Scale (Portenoy et al. 1994) as part of your assessment process. Although both instruments were originally developed for use with cancer patients, you may find them beneficial with other patient populations as well. The Edmonton and Memorial symptom assessments are available for download through the National Palliative Care Research Center (2013a, 2013b).

When assessing depression, use an appropriate clinical assessment instrument—for example, the Beck Depression Inventory or the Patient Health Questionnaire PHQ-9 (Kroenke, Spitzer, and Williams 2001). Remember to assess for suicidal ideation when assessing depression.

For information on assessing pain, the American Pain Society maintains and updates its "Clinical Practice Guidelines" online on its website (American Pain Society 2016). Also, the sixth edition of *Principles of Analgesic Use in the Treatment of Acute Pain and Cancer Pain* (American Pain Society 2008) is a valuable resource and worth consulting.

When assessing functional status, use a tool like the Palliative Performance Scale Version 2 (Victoria Hospice Society 2001), the Karnofsky Performance Scale (Cherny et al. 2015), or the Edmonton Functional Assessment Tool (Cherny et al. 2015).

For other assessment tools, check out the Palliative Care Network of Wisconsin's *Palliative Care Fast Facts* (2016) and the PEACE Project's list of assessment instruments and quality measures addressing "domains of quality of care included in the National Consensus Project for Quality Palliative Care and endorsed by the National

Quality Forum" (PEACE Project 2016). Cancer-specific guidelines for assessment can be found online through the National Comprehensive Cancer Network's website (see National Comprehensive Cancer Network 2016).

> With your relationships? With your libido (desire for sex)? With your ability to have satisfying sex with yourself or a partner?
> - What things seem to make your _____ worse?
> - What things seem to make your _____ better?
> - What do you think is causing your _____?

DIMENSION 4: DECISION MAKING

> When it comes to your health and prognosis, how direct or explicit do you want me to be? For example, if there comes a time when it seems as though you have weeks to live, would you want me to say to you, "My best guess is that you have about a week or two left to live"? or "Time is short . . . this might be a good time to begin saying your good-byes to the people closest to you"? Or would you rather I not say anything to you at all?
> - If there comes a time when you are too sick to make your wishes known regarding your care, whom do you want to make decisions on your behalf?
>   - *Have you put that decision in writing? [If the answer is yes, get a copy of the advance directive in question. If it's no, work with the patient to complete the appropriate advance directives. If you are a physician or APRN, you should discuss the issue of resuscitation preferences with the patient and complete a **do-not-resuscitate (DNR) order**, do-not-attempt-resuscitation (DNAR) order, allow-natural-death (AND) order, or **out-of-hospital provider/ physician/medical order for life-sustaining treatment (POLST/MOLST)**, as appropriate.]*

- In addition to your legal decision maker, is there anyone you would like to have involved in the shared decision-making process?
- Do you have any worries or concerns about a specific person or persons trying to step in to make decisions for you?
  - Have you discussed these concerns with that person or persons? What about with your chosen health care surrogate/decision maker?

DIMENSION 5: ANTICIPATORY PLANNING FOR DEATH

- Although it can be painful to talk about death when you are trying to focus on living, making plans for how you would like your final days to be can be a way to bring a sense of healing and peace to you and your family while you are alive.
- What would you like your surroundings to be like when you're days or hours from death?
  - Where would you like to be? In your bedroom? Somewhere else in your home? In an inpatient hospice house? Somewhere else?
  - Would you like **silence**? Music? Other sounds?
  - Are there certain scents you would like to be able to smell?
  - How would you like the room lit? Lights turned down low? Bright light from a nearby window? Soft natural light filtered through a curtain?
  - Who are the people you'd like to have at your bedside? Who would you like to have in the house but not at your bedside?
  - Are there any pets you'd like to have at your bedside?
  - Any pets you would like to have in the house but not at your bedside?
  - Would you like to have a member of the clergy or other spiritual leader at your bedside? In the house but not at your bedside?

- What would you like to be wearing? A favorite pair of pajamas? A nightshirt? Something else?
- How important is it to you that your hair and/or makeup be done in your final hours?

- Immediately after you have died, what rituals, traditions, or preferences would you like us to honor?
  - Is bathing or cleansing important to you? If so, who should be involved in the bathing/cleansing process?
  - Would you like the care team (or someone else) to change your clothes? Do you have a particular outfit you'd like your body to be dressed in?
  - Would you like friends or family to spend time at your bedside after you've died? For how long?
  - Would you like a member of the clergy or other spiritual leader to be at your bedside after you've died? For how long?
- What plans, if any, have you made for when you die?
  - Have you decided on burial, cremation, or another option?
  - Have you decided on an open casket, closed casket, or no casket?
  - Have you selected a funeral home?
  - Have you discussed plans for a funeral or memorial service with your family?
  - Would you like to have any special music, songs, hymns, religious or spiritual readings, or other passages to be included in the service?
  - Have you chosen an outfit in which to be buried or cremated?
  - Have you drafted your obituary?
  - Have you written notes or recorded videos for your family members to view after you've died?
  - Have you written an "ethical will" so that you can pass down your values to your family?
- What questions do you have about the dying process and what it may be like for someone with your illness?

DIMENSION 1B: PATIENT AS PERSON, PART 2

The purpose of Dimension 1B is to bring the assessment back to a focus on the patient as person. These questions are intended to build on the first section of the assessment, Dimension 1A, bookending the process with questions designed to elicit information and insights that will be helpful to you in meeting the patient's needs.

- When you think about your life up to this point, what are you proudest of?
- What is your biggest regret?
- What goals do you have for the remainder of your life?
- What things do you want to accomplish before you get sicker?
- What brings meaning and purpose to your life?
- What brings you joy or makes you happy?
- What brings you a feeling of control over your life?
- What are you most looking forward to in the coming days or weeks?
- What do you most want to avoid in the coming days or weeks?
- What values, beliefs, customs, and preferences would you like us to know about?
- What or who is your source of hope?
- Is there anything you're worried we might do or not do in the coming days or weeks?
- What else would you like me to know about you as a person?

ADDITIONAL QUESTIONS TO CONSIDER

The National Hospice and Palliative Care Organization (NHPCO) has outlined recommended outcomes for end-of-life care; these are reprinted in table 4.2 In the column to the right of each recommended outcome I have added questions you can ask the patient and family during your assessment, as appropriate. These questions are from the **Patient and Family Outcomes-Focused Inquiry for Developing Goals**

TABLE 4.2   PATIENT AND FAMILY OUTCOMES-FOCUSED INQUIRY
FOR DEVELOPING GOALS FOR CARE

| Domain | Recommended outcomes[a] | Patient and family outcomes-focused inquiry | |
		Questions to ask the patient	Questions to ask the family
Self-determined life closure	Staff will prevent problems associated with coping, grieving, and existential results related to imminence of death	What are your goals for coping related to the imminence of death? What are your goals for grieving related to the imminence of death? What are your goals for existential issues related to the imminence of death?	What are your goals for coping related to the imminence of death? What are your goals for grieving related to the imminence of death? What are your goals for existential issues related to the imminence of death?
	Staff will support the patient in achieving the optimal level of consciousness	How do you define your optimal level of consciousness? What are your goals for achieving the optimal level of consciousness?	How do you define the optimal level of consciousness for the patient? What are your goals for achieving the optimal level of consciousness?
	Staff will promote adaptive behaviors that are personally effective for the patient and family caregiver	What are your goals related to adaptive behaviors that are personally effective for you? What are your goals related to adaptive behaviors that are personally effective for your caregiver?	What are your goals related to adaptive behaviors that are personally effective for the patient? What are your goals related to adaptive behaviors that are personally effective for the caregiver?
Safe and comfortable dying	Staff [will] appropriately treat and prevent extension of the disease and/or comorbidity	What are your goals related to the treatment and prevention of extension of the disease and/or co-morbidity?	What are your goals related to the treatment and prevention of extension of the disease and/or co-morbidity?
	Staff [will] treat and prevent adverse effects of treatment	What are your goals related to the treatment and prevention of adverse effects of treatment?	What are your goals related to the treatment and prevention of adverse effects of treatment?

Domain	Recommended outcomes[a]	Patient and family outcomes-focused inquiry	
		Questions to ask the patient	Questions to ask the family
	Staff [will] treat and prevent distressing symptoms in concert with patient's wishes	What are your wishes regarding the treatment and prevention of distressing symptoms? What symptoms do you consider to be distressing? What are your goals related to the treatment and prevention of distressing symptoms?	What symptoms do you consider to be distressing? What are your goals related to the treatment and prevention of distressing symptoms?
	Staff [will] tailor treatments to patient's and family's functional capacity	What are your goals related to tailoring treatment to your functional capacity?	What are your goals related to tailoring treatment to your family's functional capacity? To the patient's functional capacity?
	Staff [will] prevent crises from arising due to resource deficits	What are your goals related to preventing crises from arising due to resource deficits?	What are your goals related to preventing crises from arising due to resource deficits?
	Staff [will] respond appropriately to financial, legal, and environment problems that compromise care	What are your goals related to addressing financial problems that may compromise care? What are your goals related to addressing legal problems that may compromise care? What are your goals related to addressing environment problems that may compromise care?	What are your goals related to addressing financial problems that may compromise care? What are your goals related to addressing legal problems that may compromise care? What are your goals related to addressing environment problems that may compromise care?

continued

Domain	Recommended outcomes[a]	Patient and family outcomes-focused inquiry	
		Questions to ask the patient	Questions to ask the family
Effective grieving	Staff [will] treat and prevent coping problems	What are your goals related to treating and preventing coping problems?	What are your goals related to treating and preventing coping problems in the patient?
		What are your goals related to treating and preventing your family's coping problems?	What are your goals related to treating and preventing your family's coping problems?
	Staff [will] treat and prevent adverse effects of treatment	What are your goals related to the treatment and prevention of adverse effects of treatment?	What are your goals related to the treatment and prevention of adverse effects of treatment?
	Staff [will] coach the patient and family through normal grieving	What are your goals related to being coached through normal grieving?	What are your goals related to the patient's being coached through normal grieving?
		What are your goals related to your family's being coached through normal grieving?	What are your goals related to your family's being coached through normal grieving?
	Staff [will] assess and respond to anticipatory grief	What are your goals related to staff assessing and responding to your anticipatory grief?	What are your goals related to staff assessing and responding to the patient's own anticipatory grief?
		What are your goals related to staff assessing and responding to your family's anticipatory grief?	What are your goals related to staff assessing and responding to your family's anticipatory grief?
	Staff [will] prevent unnecessary premature death	How do you define "unnecessary premature death"?	How do you define "unnecessary premature death"?
		What are your goals related to preventing unnecessary premature death?	What are your goals related to preventing unnecessary premature death?

Domain	Recommended outcomes[a]	Patient and family outcomes-focused inquiry	
		Questions to ask the patient	Questions to ask the family
	Staff [will] identify opportunities for family members' grief work	What are your goals related to identifying opportunities for your family members' grief work?	What are your goals related to identifying opportunities for your family members' grief work?
	Staff [will] assess the potential for complicated grief and respond appropriately	What are your goals related to having the staff assess and respond to complicated grief?	What are your goals related to having the staff assess and respond to complicated grief?
	Staff [will] assist the family in integrating the memory of their loved one into their lives	What are your goals for your family's integration of your memory into their lives after you've died?	What are your goals for integrating the memory of the patient into your lives after the patient has died?

Source: Institute of Medicine and National Research Council 2003.

[a] Text under "Recommended outcomes" © National Hospice and Palliative Care Organization and National Academy of Sciences. Reprinted with permission from the National Hospice and Palliative Care Organization and the National Academies Press.

for Care, a subset of the questions in the **Patient and Family Outcomes-Focused Inquiry for Interdisciplinary Teams**, which is described in Chapter 6. Use your clinical judgment regarding if, when, and how to pose these questions to patients and families during the assessment process.

DISTINGUISHING BETWEEN RELEVANT AND INTRUSIVE QUESTIONS

It is important to distinguish between questions that are relevant and necessary to your care of a patient and questions that may stem primarily from your own personal curiosity. *Transgender and gender nonconforming patients, in particular, are often subjected to intrusive questions that lack relevance to the clinical care they are seeking.* Table 4.3 lists examples of intrusive questions along with questions that are relevant to patient care.

I'd been serving as the home hospice chaplain for an eighty-year-old man, M., and his partner of forty-four years, G., for about five months when M. began the active dying process. He was brought to our hospice home, and G. kept an almost constant vigil at his bedside. G.'s sister and several friends came to sit with M. when G. had to go home to shower. During this time, my state's amendment specifically banning same-sex marriage was overturned by the Supreme Court as unconstitutional. G. and M. were suddenly able to do the unthinkable: get legally married. G. got the necessary letter from our physician indicating M. was bedbound and could not go to the county clerk's office to get the marriage license but was able to sign the letter, then G. went to that office. It happened so soon after the decision was handed down that the form still said "groom's name" and "bride's name." The clerk's office staff member had crossed out "bride" where necessary, and G. and M. had a marriage certificate.

I quickly threw together a stripped-down wedding ceremony, emphasizing the lifetime of love they had already shared and pointing out the wedding as a legal recognition of their life together. I ran to a nearby florist to get them each a boutonniere. G. came back to the hospice house and gathered his sister and a couple of dear friends. G. stood beside M.'s bed and took his hand. M. was weak and barely able to talk, but when the time came for him to speak his vows, he pledged his love in a voice strong and sure. They shared a kiss, and I had performed my first legal same-sex wedding—for men whose years together were drawing rapidly to an end. M. died just a few days later, with G. at his side, as he had been for forty-four years.

—REV. HOLLY LUX-SULLIVAN, MDIV

TABLE 4.3   RELEVANT VERSUS INTRUSIVE, CURIOSITY-DRIVEN QUESTIONS

Questions that are relevant and necessary to patient care	Intrusive questions that stem from personal curiosity
• How has your pain interfered with your libido (desire for sex)? With your ability to have satisfying sex with yourself or a partner? • Have you had any surgeries other than the ones you've already mentioned to me? What was the reason for the surgery? When did you have the surgery? Were there any complications or problems after the surgery? • What other drugs or hormones (either prescribed or obtained another way) are you currently taking? Frequency? Dose? Reason for taking? Any adverse effects? • Many people have differences or conflicts that they want to resolve before they die. What, if any, unresolved differences do you have with _____? • What sex were you assigned at birth? What gender do you identify as now? • What word or words would you use to describe your sexual orientation? What word or words would you use to describe your sexual behavior?	• How many sexual partners have you had in your lifetime? • Do you still have your penis? • Can I see your surgical scars? • When will you be "complete"? • Are your breasts "real"? • What did your parents say when you told them you were gay/lesbian/bisexual/trans? • When did you know you were gay/lesbian/bisexual/trans? • Have you ever tried having sex with someone of the other gender? • Your coming out must have been so hard for your partner. How did he/she decide to stay with you? • If you have only had sex with men, how do know you're bisexual?

THE PHYSICAL EXAMINATION

This book is intended to supplement rather than replace clinical texts. You should continue to use evidence-based best practice in conducting physical examinations of patients, congruent with your clinical discipline, licensure, and role. For example, although the following section does not include content about auscultation, you should continue to use auscultation if it is considered to be best practice for the clinical discipline in which you hold an active license and for the role you currently hold.

When performing a physical examination of a palliative care or hospice patient, physicians, APRNs, and RNs should conduct a neurological exam (including an assessment of the patient's mental status), along with a focused physical examination tailored to the individual patient's needs. Assess the patient's skin integrity and document your findings. Breast, pelvic/urogenital, rectal, and prostate exams should be performed only when appropriate and medically necessary to the care of the patient.

Patients whose birth sex does not align with their gender identity, as well as patients who have experienced sexual abuse, may feel particularly vulnerable during a physical examination. Great care should be taken to respect the privacy and dignity of every patient you examine. Explain to patients what you are going to be doing — and why — before you examine any part of their body. Encourage them to let you know if anything you are doing is causing them physical or emotional pain or discomfort.

If, during the physical exam, a patient tells you to stop or expresses pain or discomfort, *immediately stop what you're doing.* Remove your hands from the patient, take a small step back, and acknowledge (in a reassuring tone) that you heard and respect the patient's wishes. It is appropriate to ask follow-up questions, but only to the extent the patient is comfortable with them. For example, if a patient who has vulvar cancer winces when you begin the pelvic/urogenital part of the exam, it is appropriate to say (after you have stopped and moved your hands away), "I noticed that you winced when I started examining your [vulva/vagina/anus]. Can you tell me more about what you were experiencing when you winced?" Asking an open-ended question like this is better than launching immediately into a pain assessment; not all discomfort is related to physical pain.

When providing care to transgender patients, be cognizant of the fact that they may feel uncomfortable with aspects of their anatomy, whether or not those aspects are in alignment with their gender identity. A patient who was assigned the female sex at birth, currently identifies as a man, and has had **gender-affirmation surgery** may feel uncomfortable about having you see the surgical scars on his chest. A patient

who was assigned the female sex at birth, currently identifies as a man, and has chosen to affirm his gender identity
without surgical intervention may feel a sense of shame when
you examine his breasts or genitals. *No matter what anatomy
a patient has or shares with you, always treat patients according
to their gender identity.* You would never accidentally refer to a
man with gynecomastia (male breast development) as "she."
Working with transgender patients is no different. If a patient
identifies as a man, the presence of breasts (or a vagina)
doesn't change the fact he is a man and should be treated as
a man.

KEY POINTS TO REMEMBER

- To elicit a complete and accurate history from a patient,
  you need to establish a rapport with the patient and
  communicate a genuine openness to hearing the patient's
  answers to your questions.
- You can elicit the most complete and accurate history by
  using the old-school tools of the caring profession: eye
  contact, genuine listening, and a pencil and paper.
- When you take a comprehensive history of a palliative
  care or hospice patient, ask questions in each of the five
  dimensions:
  - Dimension 1A: Patient as Person, Part 1
  - Dimension 2: Illness/Treatment Summary
  - Dimension 3: Functional Activities and Symptoms
  - Dimension 4: Decision Making
  - Dimension 5: Anticipatory Planning for Death
  - Dimension 1B: Patient as Person, Part 2

- When people are diagnosed with a chronic or life-limiting
  illness, their life changes in countless ways. These
  changes can have an effect on their desire for intimacy
  with their partner or spouse. When asking questions
  about symptoms and functional abilities, remember to
  assess the impact of symptoms on sexual function.

- When taking a patient's spiritual history, be aware of the fact that that some patients may have had negative past experiences with religion. When patients are facing a chronic or life-limiting illness, they may struggle to reconcile their own spiritual beliefs with the messages they have heard from others.

DISCUSSION QUESTIONS

1. Of the five dimensions of a comprehensive history for palliative care and hospice patients, which is the most important to the delivery of high-quality care for a given patient? Which is the least important? Of the five fingers on your right hand, which is the most important to you? Which is the least important to you? How do you think these two sets of questions relate to one another?

2. Imagine that you have just met a new patient whose assigned sex at birth differs from their gender identity and expression. What are the questions that pop into your head? Which questions are relevant to your care of the patient? Which of your questions are curiosity-driven, intrusive, and not relevant to your care of the patient?

3. How much information do you need about a patient's sexual behavior in order to provide the patient with high-quality palliative or hospice care? Do you need to know about specific sexual practices? How many sexual partners the patient currently has? Whether the patient uses condoms and/or dental dams? Why or why not?

4. What are the similarities and differences between a spiritual history and a spiritual assessment in the context of palliative care and hospice?

5. Imagine you have been asked by a health care professional about your "family of origin" and your "family of choice." Who are the people you consider to be your family of origin? Who are the people you consider to be your family of choice? If you were facing a life-threatening illness, what roles would you want members of those two fami-

lies—your family of origin and your family of choice—to play in your care? How well does your family of origin know your family of choice and vice versa?

CHAPTER ACTIVITY.

Use the Five-Dimension Assessment Model to take a comprehensive history of a patient (either real or simulated via role playing). Immediately afterward, write down what you were thinking and feeling during each step in the process. Did any of your thoughts or feelings surprise you? If you used the Five-Dimension Assessment Model in your work with all patients, do you think it would improve the quality of care you deliver? Why or why not?

CHAPTER 5

SHARED DECISION MAKING AND FAMILY DYNAMICS

CHAPTER OBJECTIVES

1. Describe how you can facilitate shared decision making among the patients and families you serve.
2. Explain the ethical imperative for shared decision making.
3. Describe the process of coordinating and facilitating a family meeting focused on shared decision making.
4. Explain the role of shared decision making in palliative sedation.
5. Describe how shared decision making may be made more challenging by family dynamics for LGBTQ individuals.

Key Terms: autonomy, beneficence, ethical principles, genogram, palliative sedation, self-determination, shared decision making

Acquaviva, Kimberly
LGBTQ-Inclusive Hospice and Palliative Care
dx.doi.org/10.17312/harringtonparkpress/2017.03lgbtqihpc.005
© 2017 by Kimberly Acquaviva

Shared decision making is one of the cornerstones of quality palliative and hospice care, and it is anchored in the ethical principles of autonomy and self-determination. At its core, shared decision making is complex, and it may be made more challenging by complicated family dynamics and medically and ethically complex clinical situations. This chapter explains how to coordinate and facilitate a family meeting focused on shared decision making, how to use shared decision making for decisions surrounding **palliative sedation**, and how family dynamics may play a role in the shared decision-making process.

FACILITATING SHARED DECISION MAKING

A fundamental characteristic of both palliative care and hospice care is the central role that **shared decision making** (also referred to as "collaborative decision making") plays in the care planning process. Shared decision making is firmly rooted in the **ethical principles** of self-determination and **autonomy**: "At its core, SDM [shared decision making] rests on accepting that individual self-determination is a desirable goal and that clinicians need to support patients to achieve this goal, wherever feasible. Self-determination in the context of SDM does not mean that individuals are abandoned. SDM recognizes the need to support autonomy by building good relationships, respecting both individual competence and interdependence on others" (Elwyn et al. 2012). Regarding the historical origins of shared decision making, Stark and Fins note that it "emerged as a compromise in the longstanding debate about the relative role of patient autonomy and provider beneficence in medical decision-making" (Stark and Fins 2013).

The phrase "shared decision making" appears frequently in the literature but, as Makoul and Clayman (2006) discovered in their review of 418 articles about shared decision making, there is little agreement among health care providers as to how the concept is defined. One of the most widely cited articles about shared decision making frames the process as dyadic in nature, primarily between a physician and a patient (Charles, Gafni, and Whelan 1999). This dyadic view of shared decision making has persisted, although interdisciplinary/ interprofessional models have emerged in recent years (Sieck, Johansen, and Stewart 2016). Today there is a rich and robust body of literature on shared decision making and its use in the clinical setting (Barry and Edgman-Levitan 2012, Elwyn et al. 2014, Ferrer and Gill 2013) and a growing body of work focused on shared decision making with LGBTQ patients (DeMeester et al. 2016, Peek et al. 2016, Tan et al. 2016).

Given the interdisciplinary nature of the care provided in both palliative care and hospice settings, what does shared decision making mean within that context, and how can you facilitate the shared decision-making process? In hospice and palliative care, there are two sides to the shared decision-making equation, each of which plays an important role. On one side you have the patient and the patient's family. The patient and family bring with them their values, preferences, and goals. On the other side you have the palliative or hospice care team. The team members bring with them their knowledge, expertise, and scientific evidence. Notice that I said team rather than clinician. This is an important distinction. Each member of the interdisciplinary/interprofessional team brings to the shared decision-making process a unique perspective anchored in the evidence base of their discipline. While this collaborative, interdisciplinary approach to shared decision making may be logistically more challenging than dyadic decision making between just the patient and a single provider, patients and families are likely to benefit from the involvement of the team as a whole (Legare, Stacey, and IP Team 2014).

The text *Clinical Practice Guidelines for Quality Palliative Care* provides a detailed description of the criteria for shared decision making in its Guideline 8.1:

To assist in understanding patient and family decision-making, the patient or surrogate's expressed values, care preferences, religious beliefs, and cultural considerations are sensitively elicited, in collaboration with the family. Confirmation of these values, preferences, and considerations, with particular attention to change in health care status or transitions of care, is routinely reviewed and documented. The IDT [interdisciplinary team] discusses achievable goals for care in the context of patient values and preferences and educates the patient and family about advance care planning documents to promote communication and understanding of the patient's preferences for care across the care continuum. (National Consensus Project for Quality Palliative Care 2013)

So what does shared decision making in palliative care and hospice care look like from an operational standpoint, and which team members should be involved in the process? The answer depends in part on the decision being considered, the number of possible options, and the potential risks and benefits for the patient. Some treatment decisions—for example, the decision to put a patient who is receiving opioids on a bowel regimen—are relatively straightforward. Shared decision making regarding a bowel regimen may involve the patient and the physician, APRN, or RN, without other members of the interdisciplinary/interprofessional team. However, if a patient is reluctant to commit to following a bowel regimen, the social worker or counselor might be brought in to talk with the patient, to explore where the reluctance is coming from, and to find out whether preventing constipation is one of the patient's goals.

Other treatment decisions, such as decisions regarding the management of delirium in a patient nearing the end of life, may be more complex and necessitate the involvement of multiple team members in the shared decision-making process. It's worth emphasizing, however, that all members of the interdisciplinary/interprofessional team share responsibility, within each member's scope of practice, for helping patients achieve all of their goals.

SHARED DECISION-MAKING SCENARIO

Let's use a fictional case involving a patient with delirium to illustrate the shared decision-making process and the role of each member of the interdisciplinary team. While the treatment of delirium might be viewed as a strictly medical issue, there may be psychosocial and spiritual components of relevance to the decision-making process. As Ross and Alexander (2001) write: "Hospice workers have noted that a changed mental status is more pronounced in patients who have been undergoing a significant psychosocial or spiritual struggle. They would argue that sedation is not appropriate in this setting. For families, however, the open, staring eyes and agitated movement of a patient may not be emotionally tolerable, resulting in a request for something to 'quiet' the patient."

Given that delirium may be seen near the end of life and that it can be emotionally upsetting for families to witness, shared decisions regarding its treatment may involve the patient's family (as defined by the patient), the physician, APRN, RN, social worker, counselor, and/or chaplain, especially when palliative sedation is being considered as a treatment option.

ABOUT THE PATIENT AND FAMILY

In our scenario, the patient experiencing delirium is a fifty-six-year-old woman named Mary. Mary received palliative care for two years while she was seeking curative treatment for ovarian cancer. Mary transitioned from palliative care to in-home hospice care two weeks ago and, after a precipitous decline, she now appears to be days from death. Her partner of twenty years and primary caregiver, Martha, is very distressed by Mary's delirium. Five years ago, Mary named Martha her durable power of attorney for health care.

WHAT IS PALLIATIVE SEDATION?

- "Palliative sedation is the monitored use of medications intended to induce varying degrees of unconsciousness, but not death, for relief of refractory and unendurable symptoms in imminently dying patents." (Dahlin and Lynch 2003)
- "Palliative sedation is a treatment of last resort when symptom distress cannot be relieved using standard methods. It is used extremely rarely because the vast majority of patients get acceptable relief without sedation." (Center to Advance Palliative Care 2010)
- "Palliative sedation . . . is the intentional lowering of awareness towards, and including, unconsciousness for patients with severe and refractory symptoms." (American Academy of Hospice and Palliative Medicine 2014)
- "There is no clear consensus or scientific evidence regarding the most appropriate medication(s) to effect palliative sedation. As elsewhere in medicine, the agent should be selected based on safety, efficacy, and availability." (American Academy of Hospice and Palliative Medicine 2014)

Because of the intense need for round-the-clock **symptom management** in the past several days, the hospice team has put continuous-care RNs in place. Martha keeps asking the nurses to "do something" because she's worried that Mary is in pain. After searching online for information on ways to help Mary, Martha expresses interest in palliative sedation.

Mary's mother and father, estranged from Mary since she left home at age eighteen, are also at the bedside. Martha called Mary's parents a week ago because Mary said she wanted a chance to tell them good-bye. At that time, Mary was still alert and communicating clearly, and she didn't appear to be in any distress. When Mary's parents arrived, they told Mary they loved her but they were suffering deeply because they believed she was going to "burn in the fires of hell" if she didn't "accept Jesus Christ as her Lord and Savior" before she died. Mary tried to change the subject to something that wasn't so contentious, but her parents were adamant: they said if she didn't get "saved" before she died, she would suffer eternal damnation. In the days following, Mary's level of consciousness changed, she stopped speaking, and she began intermittently moaning and thrashing.

Mary's parents are now convinced that her current distress is a sign that she's "trying to get right with the Lord" before she dies. For this reason, they are insisting that they don't want Mary to be sedated, and they have repeatedly asserted that, as Mary's parents, they should have been appointed as her legal decision makers. Martha (Mary's legal decision maker) does not share Mary's parents' belief about the cause of Mary's distress, and she feels strongly that Mary should be sedated to relieve her agitation. Martha says Mary told her many times that she wanted Martha to do whatever she could to make sure Mary didn't "suffer" in her last days.

WHO ARE THE DECISION MAKERS?

In this scenario, there are four individuals (the patient, the patient's partner, and the patient's two parents) whose needs the hospice interdisciplinary team must try to meet. Of central concern is Mary, the patient. Since Mary is unable to participate in the shared decision-making process owing to her delirium, her partner, Martha—who was appointed Mary's durable power of attorney for health care—is the individual with the legal right to make decisions on Mary's behalf. After their long period of estrangement, Mary's parents are seeking to reengage with their daughter, but their religious beliefs and lack of understanding about Martha's decision-making rights are causing distress—for Martha as well as for themselves. Although Martha is legally the decision maker, involving Mary's parents in the shared decision-making process to the extent that Martha is comfortable may help to decrease the emotional distress for all the parties involved.

Although Mary did not explicitly express her desire for palliative sedation prior to her recent decline, she told her partner (her legal decision maker) about her wishes regarding the alleviation of suffering at the end of life. Her preferences should drive the decision-making process: "While it seems an ethical imperative to involve family members and other persons close to the patient when identifying the values of a patient lacking capacity or, where relevant, to interpret any advance statement in terms of the decision about palliative sedation therapy, the role of family members as decision makers is restricted to those legally representing the patient. Even in such a case it seems important to stress that family members or other people who have taken up this task as representatives must base their decisions on the (presumed) will of the patient" (Schildmann and Schildmann 2014). Martha's advocacy for Mary is clearly anchored in what she believes to be the will of the patient, Mary.

FACILITATING THE SHARED DECISION-MAKING PROCESS

There are almost infinite possibilities for how the interdisciplinary team could facilitate the shared decision-making process in this case. The following scenario describes just one way the team might choose to proceed.

Team Discussion about Ethics, Risks, and Benefits

At the hospice interdisciplinary team meeting, the social worker raises the issue of Mary's delirium and asks the other team members for their thoughts regarding the possibility of using palliative sedation to alleviate Mary's delirium. The RN says that, since Mary seems to be imminently dying and other efforts to manage her symptoms have been unsuccessful in addressing her delirium, palliative sedation seems like an appropriate option to explore and would be consistent with the Hospice and Palliative Nurses Association's "Position Statement: Palliative Sedation at End of Life" (Dahlin and Lynch 2003). The physician agrees and adds that, because Mary is no longer eating or drinking, no longer substantially interacting with those around her, and no longer making decisions regarding her own care, palliative sedation does not seem to raise any ethical concerns from her perspective (which is consistent with American Academy of Hospice and Palliative Medicine's "Palliative Sedation Position Statement"; see AAHPM 2014). The physician conveys to the team that, in her professional opinion, the use of palliative sedation to treat Mary's delirium would meet AAHPM's four criteria for ethical defensibility (AAHPM 2014):

1. Palliative sedation will be used only "after careful interdisciplinary evaluation and treatment of the patient."
2. "Palliative treatments that are not intended to affect consciousness have failed or, in the judgment of the clinician, are very likely to fail."
3. The use of palliative sedation "is not expected to shorten the patient's time to death."
4. Palliative sedation will be used "only for the actual or expected duration of symptoms."

After hearing the physician read off this list of criteria, the RN comments on how different the AAHPM and HPNA (Hospice and Palliative Nurses Association) positions are regarding when palliative sedation is ethically defensible. According to the HPNA:

> The use of medication to promote comfort and relieve pain in dying patients is supported by the American Nurses Association (ANA) . . . , [which states that] "achieving adequate symptom control, even at the expense of life, thus hastening death is ethically justified." This statement is reiterated in the ANA's

Code of Ethics for Nurses[,] which also states that nurses may not act with the sole intent to end a patient's life even if motivated by compassion and concern for dignity and quality of life. Thus, palliative sedation with its intent to relieve suffering in dying patients but not to deliberately hasten death is seen as distinct from euthanasia or assisted suicide where the intent is solely to end life. These statements reflect the rule of double effect. (Dahlin and Lynch 2003)

After a brief discussion about the evidence in the literature, both the RN and the physician agree that there does not appear to be a risk that palliative sedation would hasten Mary's death. Given that palliative sedation appears to be both clinically appropriate and ethically defensible, the team physician is supportive of palliative sedation and says she will contact Mary's primary care physician immediately after the meeting to discuss moving the plan forward, assuming the rest of the team agrees this is the appropriate course of action. The team social worker expresses concern about the tension and conflict between Mary's parents and Martha, and worries aloud that Mary's parents will become even more agitated if Mary is sedated. The team chaplain echoes the social worker's concerns and indicates that she is planning to visit the patient and family later that day to provide spiritual support. The chaplain adds that she suspects Mary's agitation stems from the frightening message of damnation that her parents repeatedly conveyed to her. The interdisciplinary team as a whole comes to consensus that the shared decision-making process needs to begin with a conversation between the hospice physician, registered nurse, social worker, chaplain, Martha, and Mary's parents. (Martha had previously expressed that she wasn't interested in meeting one on one with the chaplain, but she was supportive of the idea of the chaplain supporting Mary's parents.)

In preparation for engaging in the shared decision-making process with Mary's partner and parents, the interdisciplinary team discusses the different dimensions of palliative sedation as a potential treatment for Mary's delirium, using something like the chart shown as table 5.1. Working from left to right, the team discusses each dimension and rates its level of potential risk or benefit. Table 5.1 is a template; table 5.2 shows a chart as completed by the team in the case study.

Quantifying the potential risks and benefits of a given treatment option is an evidence-based endeavor and should be grounded in the literature to the extent possible. Because each member of the interdisciplinary team is familiar with a different body of literature (namely, the one anchored in their own discipline), disagreements may occur among team members about perceived degrees of risk or benefit along the various dimensions. The team members do not need to reach perfect consensus on the degrees of risk and benefit. What is important is that the members of the team have an open discussion about each dimension so that, when they meet with the patient and family, they have a shared understanding of how they plan to present the risks and benefits of a given treatment option.

Coordination with the Primary Care Provider
After the interdisciplinary team meeting, the hospice physician reaches out to Mary's primary care physician to begin discussing the possibility of palliative sedation. The primary care physician is supportive of the hospice physician's recommendation that palliative sedation be used to address Mary's delirium.

Setting Up the Family Meeting
After the hospice physician gets off the phone with Mary's primary care physician, she contacts the team social worker to request assistance with setting up a meeting at the patient's home later that day. The team social worker calls the team nurse and they find a block of time that works for all of the team members, including the chaplain. The social worker

TABLE 5.1 **RISK-BENEFIT DISCUSSION TOOL FOR SHARED DECISION MAKING IN HOSPICE AND PALLIATIVE CARE**

Risk of exacerbation of physical symptoms	minimal	low	moderate	high
Potential for alleviation of physical symptoms	minimal	low	moderate	high
Risk of negative impact on quality of life	minimal	low	moderate	high
Potential for positive impact on quality of life	minimal	low	moderate	high
Risk of shortening length of life	minimal	low	moderate	high
Potential for extending length of life	minimal	low	moderate	high
Risk of exacerbation of psychosocial and/or spiritual issues	minimal	low	moderate	high
Potential for alleviation of psychosocial and/or spiritual issues	minimal	low	moderate	high

TABLE 5.2 **COMPLETED RISK-BENEFIT DISCUSSION TOOL FOR SHARED DECISION MAKING IN HOSPICE AND PALLIATIVE CARE**

Risk of exacerbation of physical symptoms	**minimal**	low	moderate	high
Potential for alleviation of physical symptoms	minimal	low	moderate	**high**
Risk of negative impact on quality of life	**minimal**	low	moderate	high
Potential for positive impact on quality of life	**minimal**	low	moderate	high
Risk of shortening length of life	minimal	**low**	moderate	high
Potential for extending length of life	**minimal**	low	moderate	high
Risk of exacerbation of psychosocial and/or spiritual issues	**minimal** for patient	low	**moderate** for parents	high
Potential for alleviation of psychosocial and/or spiritual issues	minimal	low	**moderate** for partner	high

The extent to which interdisciplinary team members other than the physician have real decision-making power regarding the use of palliative sedation for a given patient is unclear. As Schildmann and Schildmann discovered in their analysis of eight sets of guidelines on palliative sedation: "Guidelines on [palliative sedation therapy] differ also with regards to recommendations on the appropriate roles of the different health care professionals in decision making. The majority of guidelines recommend involvement of nonphysician health care professionals. . . . While a consensus within the multiprofessional palliative care team in practice seems important especially in difficult situations of end-of-life care, it is not clear in the majority of guidelines how the stakeholders should proceed in the case of disagreement" (Schildmann and Schildmann 2014).

Within your palliative care service or hospice program, find out whether guidelines are in place for how decision making and disagreements are handled with regard to palliative sedation. Your palliative care or hospice program may have an ethics committee that consults on challenging cases, such as those involving palliative sedation. When does the ethics committee get involved in a case, and what triggers its involvement? Can any member of the interdisciplinary team request an ethics consult? If no guidelines currently exist in your organization, talk with the medical director to express an interest in being part of an interdisciplinary effort to develop them, then offer to take the lead on coordinating the effort. Physicians, APRNs, RNs, chaplains, social workers, counselors, and pharmacists are ideally suited to work collaboratively— and proactively—to develop guidelines to smooth the way for their future interactions around difficult decisions like palliative sedation.

calls Martha, confirms that the time works for her as well as for Mary's parents, and briefly explains the purpose of the meeting. During the call, the social worker reiterates that the hospice team recognizes Martha as Mary's legal decision maker, and explains that the chaplain will be coming to provide support for Mary's parents if Martha is comfortable with that. Martha says she's open to the chaplain's involvement if it will be helpful to Mary's parents.

The Family Meeting
At the designated time, the hospice physician, registered nurse, social worker, and chaplain arrive at Mary and Martha's home. When Martha opens the front door, her eyes are puffy and red from crying. It looks like Mary's parents have been crying as well. The social worker asks Martha where she would feel most comfortable meeting with the team. Martha asks whether the meeting can take place in the room where Mary is, "so that it feels like she's part of the decision." Mary's mother says she'd like that—she doesn't want to leave Mary's bedside. The registered nurse, physician, social worker, and chaplain pull up chairs around Mary's bed so that everyone is seated in a circle around her. Because the RN is the team member who has formed the strongest bond with the patient and family in the short time the patient has been receiving hospice care, the nurse starts off the meeting. The RN explains that the purpose of the meeting is to discuss options for making sure Mary is as comfortable as possible. The nurse frames the purpose of the meeting this way because ensuring Mary's comfort is the one thing that Martha and Mary's parents agree on. Thus, the RN helps to lay the foundation for a shared decision-making session in which Martha and Mary's parents can work together toward that common goal.

The social worker asks Martha and Mary's parents what their goal or hope is for Mary's final days. Martha says her goal is for Mary "to be able to die peacefully without so much suffering." Mary's father says his hope is for his daughter to "be able to die a Christian." At hearing this, Mary's mother nods and begins weeping. The chaplain says gently that she thinks the hospice team can help Martha and Mary's parents ensure that Mary's final days are as peaceful as possible. She says that even though Mary is no longer speaking, her parents can pray for her and help Mary resolve unfinished business that may be causing her some distress. The chaplain suggests that four of the greatest gifts parents can give their dying child are unconditional love, apologies, forgiveness, and permission. The chaplain lets a brief silence hang in the air. Mary's father asks the chaplain how to do that. The chaplain tells Mary's father and mother that there is no right or wrong way; the main idea is to:

1. Tell Mary that they love her the way she is — she doesn't need to change anything to be worthy of their love;
2. Tell Mary that they're sorry for any hurt they may have caused her over the years;
3. Tell Mary that they forgive her for any hurt she may have caused them over the years; and
4. Tell Mary that it's all right for her to let go — she doesn't need to hang on for them.

On hearing the chaplain's words, Mary's parents visibly soften and Mary's father begins to weep. The hospice team sits with the family, providing a silent, supportive presence. After several minutes, the physician brings the issue of Mary's delirium into the conversation. She explains what delirium is and describes the treatments for Mary's delirium that have been tried so far. She asks first Martha and then Mary's parents how Mary's delirium is affecting them. All three agree that Mary's delirium is extremely upsetting to them and that being at Mary's bedside is, as Mary's father puts it, "almost more painful than not being there at all." The physician asks Martha whether she can think of anything that might be causing Mary's distress. Martha says that her distress seemed to have started when Mary's parents arrived and began telling her she was going to go to hell when she died if she didn't accept Jesus before it was too late. Martha quickly turns to Mary's parents and says she's not trying to blame them—she knows they were just doing what they thought was best for their daughter. Martha pauses and then adds, "I wish you knew Mary like I do. She is the kindest, most compassionate human being you could ever imagine. If Mary's going to hell, there's not much hope for anybody." Martha begins to weep. Mary's mother reaches over tentatively and puts her arm around Martha's shoulder in support.

Next, the physician explains palliative sedation as an option for treating Mary's delirium. Using the risk-benefit chart that the interdisciplinary team explored prior to the family meeting, the physician walks Martha and Mary's parents through the potential risks and benefits of palliative sedation (see table 5.2). She talks about each dimension in the chart and asks questions of both Martha and Mary's parents to make sure they all understand the information she is presenting. When the physician gets to the assessment of the risk of shortening the length of Mary's life, Mary's parents say they are relieved to hear that palliative sedation isn't euthanasia— they say that before the meeting, they had thought "palliative sedation" was synonymous with "euthanasia." The physician affirms that this is a common misconception and that scientific evidence supports the finding that palliative sedation, when used appropriately, does not hasten death (Maltoni et al. 2009).

After hearing about all of the potential risks and benefits, Martha says she thinks she wants to move forward with sedating Mary but she's not sure. Martha turns to Mary's parents and says she would like to have their help in making this difficult decision. Mary's father asks whether it would be possible for them to have some time "to say the things that need to be said" before Mary is sedated, if sedation is what Martha decides is the right thing to do. Martha nods and says she thinks that is a good idea. Mary's mother thanks Martha for being willing to do that. Martha turns to the hospice physician and says she would like to move forward with palliative sedation for Mary, starting the following morning. Martha signs an **informed consent** form for the palliative sedation. The hospice physician (working in concert with the primary care physician) arranges for a prescription of continuous subcutaneous midazolam to be delivered to the home later that day. The plan is for the medication to be carefully titrated and Mary to be carefully monitored to ensure that a deep level of sedation in maintained (Periyakoil n.d.). As the hospice social worker wraps up the meeting with the family, Mary's father asks if the chaplain can stay for a while. The chaplain agrees and the rest of the team leaves. A registered nurse remains in the home to provide continuous care.

That afternoon, the chaplain sits with Mary's parents at the bedside. Mary's parents pray with the chaplain and tell Mary all the things they wish they had said to her before she got sick. They tell her they're proud of her and that they see what a kind person Martha is. They apologize for saying hurtful things to Mary over the years, and they forgive Mary for the hurtful things she said to them. They tell Mary that it's okay for her to let go when she's ready. They tell Mary that they will do their best to support Martha in her grief, and that they know Martha will do the same for them. Most important, they tell Mary that they love her unconditionally.

Ultimately Mary did not need to be sedated. Shortly after Mary's parents spoke to her at her bedside, Mary's delirium decreased significantly and she began resting comfortably. Mary died less than twenty-four hours later.

SHARED DECISION-MAKING SCENARIO DEBRIEFING

Reading this scenario, you may be thinking to yourself that in "real life" the hospice physician, registered nurse, social worker, and chaplain would never make a joint home visit for the purpose of shared decision making. How could a hospice program afford to send four members of an interdisciplinary team to a single patient's home for an hour-long shared decision-making session? Wouldn't it be more efficient to have just the physician or RN meet with a family caregiver like Martha? And since the hospice team did not even end up using palliative sedation, what was the point of this whole scenario?

I used this scenario because it illustrates how complicated shared decision making can be even when it's done well. Shared decision making is not easy or efficient. It takes time and effort to walk a patient and family through the options available to them, and sometimes the only real "intervention" you end up providing is the shared decision-making session itself. In the scenario I just described, four interdisciplinary team members spent fifteen minutes in a meeting prior to the visit and sixty minutes during the visit on the shared decision-making process. Five person-hours (plus travel time) were spent facilitating the shared decision making regarding Mary's delirium. In the grand scheme of things, this is not a large investment of time.

In the scenario described, there were complex family dynamics and spiritual/existential concerns. Had those factors not been understood and addressed by the team as a whole, the spiritual distress Mary's parents felt and the emotional distress experienced by Martha might have worsened, and then the conflict in the home would have been exacerbated by the decision to move forward with palliative sedation. By working collaboratively with the patient and her family, the interdisciplinary team was able to give Martha and Mary's parents the tools they needed to alleviate Mary's suffering—and their own.

FAMILY DYNAMICS AND SHARED DECISION MAKING

According to Bowen family systems theory, the family is "an emotional unit" that "so profoundly affect[s] their members' thoughts, feelings, and actions that it often seems as if people are living under the same 'emotional skin'" (Kerr 2000). Kerr explains: "People solicit each other's attention, approval, and support and react to each other's needs, expectations, and upsets. The connectedness and reactivity make the functioning of family members interdependent. A change in one person's functioning is predictably followed by reciprocal changes in the functioning of others. Families differ somewhat in the degree of interdependence, but it is always present to some degree."

Sometimes an individual will try to reduce the tension associated with interacting with their family by using a strategy Bowen family systems theory calls "emotional cutoff": "The concept of emotional cut off describes people managing their unresolved emotional issues with parents, siblings, and other family members by reducing or totally cutting off emotional contact with them. Emotional contact can be reduced by people moving away from their families and rarely going home, or it can be reduced by people staying in physical contact with their families but avoiding sensitive issues. Relationships may look 'better' if people cut off to manage them, but the problems are dormant and not resolved" (Kerr 2000).

As a palliative care or hospice care provider, you are likely to encounter patients who have been cut off emotionally from their families of origin, either voluntarily through their own actions or involuntarily through the actions of their family members. In the scenario presented in this chapter, two families—Mary's family of origin and her family of choice—came together at her bedside during an emotionally difficult time, each bringing a unique set of family dynamics that governed the families' respective interactions with Mary. To manage the tension surrounding Mary's sexual orientation and her parents' evangelical Christian religious beliefs, Mary and her parents had cut off contact with each other years before. The issues between them resurfaced as Mary was dying, leading to distress for the patient, her partner, and her parents.

Although you may see estrangement in families of LGBTQ individuals in palliative and hospice care, you are also likely to see it in the families of heterosexual and cisgender people (Lawton, White, and Fromme 2014; Mazanec and Panke 2016). When you are working with LGBTQ patients, don't assume that their parents have disowned them, judged them, or shunned them, and don't assume they have not. The same holds true when you are working with heterosexual or cisgender patients: do not make any assumptions about patients' relationships with their families of origin. Families are like snowflakes: no two are exactly the same. The only way to know what the dynamics in a particular patient's family are like is to ask the patient. Ask not only who their legal decision maker is (e.g., the person they have appointed to serve as their durable power of attorney for health care or is their health care proxy) but also about who they would like to have included—and excluded—from discussions surrounding decisions about their care.

AUTHOR'S NOTE

My own family is a good example of why you should never make assumptions about a patient's family and the roles of those family members in the shared decision-making process. My mom and dad were a legally married, deeply religious couple, and I was their lesbian daughter living thousands of miles away. It would have been easy to make assumptions about my family and the roles that each of us would play in the decision-making process if one of my parents became ill, but those assumptions would have been wrong. When my mother was dying, I was in my mid-twenties, living in Philadelphia. I went home to Texas to help my father take care of her during the last six weeks of her life.

Because my parents were married, my dad would have been the default decision maker for my mother's health care decisions. However, my mom had named me as her durable power of attorney (DPOA) for health care because she didn't want my dad to have the burden of making tough decisions about things like forgoing artificial nutrition and hydration. My dad was fully supportive of my mom's decision to name me as the DPOA for health care, but he wanted to remain involved in the decision-making process—and I really needed his involvement. When my mom became unable to make her own health care decisions, I made those decisions in consultation with my dad, and I made sure that he had a voice in all decisions that were made. Working together, my dad and I were able to ensure that my mom died comfortably and without any futile extraordinary measures. Unfortunately my mom was on hospice care for only a few days before she died—a common problem. Often patients get referred to hospice care far too late in the progression of their illness. Had my mom been on hospice care for a longer time, the hospice team would likely have played a role in supporting our family's shared decision-making efforts.

MAPPING FAMILY DYNAMICS

When you begin working with a new patient, make note of any distinguishing features of the patient's relationships with members of their family of origin and family of choice. Creating a **genogram** is one way to map the emotional relationships within a patient's family constellation. Inexpensive software programs like GenoPro can help you create a genogram quickly and easily, but you can also compile a genogram using pen and paper. (If you decide to use GenoPro, be aware that the program's "rules to build a genogram" have a heterosexist bias: "In the case of ambiguity, assume a male-female relationship, rather than male-male or female-female relationship" [GenoPro 2016b].) When indicating that a patient or family member is male or female in a genogram, record the person's gender identity rather than biological or anatomical sex.

Whether or not you draw up a genogram, take the time to ask patients about the different emotional relationships in their family of origin and family of choice, and the communication patterns between the two (Smolinski and Colón 2011). This information will be incredibly helpful to you as you work to support patients and families and facilitate effective shared decision making.

- A fundamental characteristic of both palliative care and hospice care is the central role that shared decision making plays in the care-planning process.
- Shared decision making is firmly rooted in the ethical principles of self-determination and autonomy.
- In hospice and palliative care, shared decision making is a two-sided equation, with the patient and family on one side and the palliative care or hospice care team on the other.
- Shared decision making is not easy or efficient. It takes time and effort to walk a patient and family through the options available to them, and sometimes the only real "intervention" you end up providing is the shared decision-making session itself.
- When working with LGBTQ patients, do not assume that their parents disowned them, judged them, or shunned them. Do not assume they didn't, either. When working with heterosexual or cisgender patients, the same holds true: do not make any assumptions about their relationships with their families of origin.
- The only way to know what the dynamics are like within a particular patient's family is to ask the patient. Ask questions not only about who will be the legal decision maker (i.e., who has their durable power of attorney for health care or their health care proxy) but also about who they would like to have included—and excluded—from discussions surrounding their health care decisions.
- When you begin working with a new patient, make note of any distinguishing features of the patient's relationship with members of their family of origin and their family of choice. Creating a genogram is one way to do this. Regardless of whether you draw a genogram, always ask

the patient about the different emotional relationships in their family of origin and family of choice.

DISCUSSION QUESTIONS

1. Why is it important to think of the first patient encounter as a "family meeting," even if the patient decides not to include family members in the visit?

2. Describe how you would coordinate and facilitate a family meeting focused on shared decision making, starting from your very first meeting with the patient.

3. What role do ethics play in shared decision making? Explain the ethical imperative for shared decision making.

4. Explain the role of shared decision making in decisions surrounding palliative sedation. What role does your own discipline play in those decisions? If a patient expressed interest in palliative sedation, how do you think you would feel? How would you respond?

5. How might shared decision making be made more challenging by family dynamics for LGBTQ individuals?

CHAPTER ACTIVITY

Draw a genogram of the emotional relationships in your family, including members of both your family of origin and your family of choice. You can find a comprehensive list of connector symbols for use in representing the emotional relationships between individuals online at http://www.genopro.com/genogram/emotional-relationships/. After you have drawn your genogram, reflect on what the diagram reveals about the relationships in your family. Would these emotional relationships be immediately apparent to a health care professional who had just met you? Would having an understanding of these relationships be helpful to a palliative care or hospice professional caring for you? Why or why not?

CHAPTER 6

CARE PLANNING AND COORDINATION

CHAPTER OBJECTIVES

1. Describe how to help patients and their families formulate and track progress toward goals of care and expected outcomes.

2. List questions that interdisciplinary/interprofessional team members can ask one another during team meetings to keep the plan of care focused on patient- and family-centered outcomes.

3. Describe how to assess for environmental and safety risks and provide suggestions for modifying a patient's environment to minimize safety risks.

Key Terms: environmental and safety assessment, expected outcomes, goals of care, Patient and Family Outcomes-Focused Inquiry for Interdisciplinary Teams, plan of care

Acquaviva, Kimberly
LGBTQ-Inclusive Hospice and Palliative Care
dx.doi.org/10.17312/harringtonparkpress/2017.03lgbtqihpc.006
© 2017 by Kimberly Acquaviva

In palliative care and hospice care, the patient and family (as defined by the patient) are the unit of care, and the plan of care is focused on the patient's and family's goals of care. Helping patients and families identify their own goals requires both skill and a commitment to avoiding the temptation to use the "drop-down menu" goals of care provided in many electronic health records. This chapter explains how to help patients and families identify their own unique goals, how to use a set of key questions to refocus interdisciplinary/interprofessional team meetings on patient- and family-centered outcomes of care, and how to conduct an environmental and safety risk assessment.

In Chapter 5 we explored the concept and practice of shared decision making. While it may seem odd to place the chapter about setting goals of care *after* the chapter on shared decision making, this sequence is intentional. Your work with patients and families is not strictly linear or sequential—care planning and shared decision making occur contemporaneously; the two concepts are inextricably intertwined. However, having an understanding of shared decision making is foundational to understanding care planning and coordination.

PLAN OF CARE

When a patient begins receiving palliative care or hospice care, the **interdisciplinary/interprofessional team** puts together a **plan of care** built around the patient's and family's goals. The Five-Dimension Assessment Model (presented in detail in Chapter 4) provides a comprehensive list of LGBTQ-inclusive questions for use during the history-taking process, designed to help elicit the patient's and family's goals of care. In addition to the patient's and family's goals, the plan of care, developed after a "comprehensive and timely interdisciplinary assessment of the patient and family," should take into account "the patient's current medical status; adequacy of diagnosis and treatment consistent with review of past history; diagnosis and treatment; and responses to past treatments," as well as "documentation of disease status; diagnoses and prognosis; comorbid medical and psychiatric disorders; physical and psychological symptoms; functional status; social, cultural, and spiritual strengths, values, practices, concerns, and goals; advance care planning concerns, preferences, and documents; and [for palliative care patients,] appropriateness of hospice referral" (National Consensus Project for Quality Palliative Care 2013).

Other essential elements of the care plan include documenting the ways in which the patient and family understand the patient's illness, including their "expectations of treatment, goals for care, quality of life, . . . [and] preferences for the type and site of care." Equally important to the care planning process is identifying "the elements of quality of life" in the physical, social, spiritual, and psychological domains and then planning interventions "to alleviate stress in one or any of these domains." The result of the care planning process is a "care plan . . . based on the identified and expressed preferences, values, goals, and needs of the patient and family and . . . developed with professional guidance and support for patient/family decision making" (National Consensus Project for Quality Palliative Care 2013). By design, the care plan is not static and unchanging, nor is its development the work of the interdisciplinary team (IDT) alone. On the contrary:

> The care plan is based upon an ongoing assessment and reflects goals set by the patient, family or surrogate in collaboration with the IDT. Such goals reflect the changing benefits and burdens of various care options, at critical decision points during the course of illness. In collaboration with the patient, family, and other involved health care professionals, the IDT develops the care plan with the additional input, when indicated, from other community providers such as school professionals, community service providers, and spiritual leaders. Changes in the care plan are based on the evolving needs and

preferences of the patient and family, with recognition of the complex, competing, and shifting priorities in goals of care. The evolving care plan is documented over time. (National Consensus Project for Quality Palliative Care 2013)

GOALS OF CARE AND EXPECTED OUTCOMES

The patient's and family's goals of care and their **expected outcomes** serve as the cornerstones for each plan of care. Goals of care are straightforward, simple statements aligned with the hopes, values, priorities, and fears expressed by the patient and family (Vermont Ethics Network 2011c). Once you have helped a patient or family member identify a goal, ask follow-up questions that will help them articulate what the successful achievement or outcome of that goal would look like. For example, Mr. Smith might express one of his goals as, "I want to get a good night's sleep." Your follow-up questions to Mr. Smith might be:

- What does "a good night's sleep" mean to you? (Mr. Smith's answer: "Six hours without waking up.")
- Are you having trouble falling asleep, staying asleep, or both? (Mr. Smith's answer: "Staying asleep.")
- Is anything in particular waking you up? (Mr. Smith's answer: "Pain—the pain wakes me up every time.")

Expected outcomes—the outcomes of your interventions toward achieving the goal—should be measurable and time-limited; they should state what will happen, and when. To develop an expected outcome aligned with Mr. Smith's goal of a good night's sleep, for example, put together the following components (Austin Community College n.d.):

- a subject ("Mr. Smith")
- a verb in future tense ("will sleep")
- a condition ("without pain waking him up")
- a criterion ("for at least six consecutive hours")
- a time ("tonight")

TABLE 6.1 EXAMPLES OF EXPECTED OUTCOMES

Subject	Verb (future tense)	Condition	Criteria	Time
Mr. Smith (the patient)	will sleep	without pain waking him up	for at least six consecutive hours	tonight
Mr. Jones (Mr. Smith's partner)	will attend his Thursday twelve-step meeting	with respite care in the home for Mr. Smith	for two hours (6:00 pm–8:00 pm)	this Thursday
Mr. Smith (the patient)	will urinate	without falling	using a bedside commode	tonight

Here is how Mr. Smith's goal and expected outcome might align:

Patient's goal: To sleep soundly.

Expected outcome: Mr. Smith will sleep, without pain waking him up, for at least six consecutive hours tonight.

Table 6.1 provides a few other examples of expected outcomes.

As goals of care change over time, your task is to collaborate with the patient, family, and other members of the interdisciplinary/interprofessional team to modify the plan of care to facilitate achieving the revised goals and expected outcomes. If you have been working in the field of palliative care or hospice for a few years, you may have noticed that you are writing down similar goals for care for most of your patients: "live independently," "remain as pain-free as possible," "achieve remission or cure" (for palliative care patients), "spend quality time with family and friends," and so on.

While there are certainly some naturally occurring commonalities among patients and families regarding goals of care, you should try to identify some unique goals for each patient and family you work with. It's easy to fall into a rut, charting the same goals of care over and over again, especially if you use an electronic health record that includes a menu of often-cited goals. Resist the urge to take shortcuts when it comes to goals of care.

One of the most memorable patients that I took care of in palliative care and subsequently in hospice was a gay man with HIV/AIDS who willfully decided to stop taking antiretroviral therapy because he was "fed up with the world" and "ready to die." The biggest challenge in taking care of him was establishing good rapport. He was mistrustful of the health care system at large, owing to feelings of abandonment and judgment. As an advocate and provider [of] LGBTQ medicine, I only wanted what was best for this population, [which] collectively has been pushed to the sidelines and not necessarily receive[d] the best quality of care afforded to the general population. One night in the hospice unit, as he was dying, it was found out that not even his mother, his only known family, knew of his illness. Up to the last few moments of his life, he felt alone. I took refuge in hospice being there for him and in a sense became a surrogate support. I was moved by images of a mother grieving and crying at the bedside and a son who felt betrayed by society. I felt like there was a hint of vindication in that he at least received the best medical and psychosocial care possible at that stage of his life. But did he really? The truth is that there continue to be gaps in knowledge and skills in taking care of the palliative care and hospice needs of the seriously ill in this population.

—NOELLE MARIE C. JAVIER, MD

When I first started working with patients struggling with serious or life-limiting illnesses, I had the good fortune to work with mentors who encouraged me to craft patient- and family-specific goals of care in collaboration with the

It's important to take the time to search for goals that people are actually motivated to achieve and start there. For example, a person might say that she injured her back and "wishes she had help." As the health care provider, we might say then that the goal is to get caregiver assistance. The patient might reply, "John would never allow anyone in the house but our daughter, and she has not been speaking to us lately." Our response: "Would you be willing/able to give her a call to speak with her about it?" Patient's response: "John might not like that." Our response: "Could you speak with John about it?" Patient's response: "Yes."

So the goal is not to get a caregiver. The goal is for the patient to speak to her husband about possibilities. All too often we jump to "our end goal," setting people up for the dreaded "noncompliant" label by continuing to ask them, "Have you gotten a caregiver yet?" — overlooking the critical first steps . . . and setting them up for failure.

—GARY GARDIA, M.ED, MSW, LCSW

patient, family, and the rest of the interdisciplinary/interprofessional team. The piece that was missing, though, was a tool to help me brainstorm a broad range of goals with the patient and family, inclusive of their sexual orientation, gender identity, and sexual health.

Almost twenty years later we still don't have a comprehensive tool like that for use by palliative care and hospice teams. With the wide variety of electronic health records in use, proposing a one-size-fits-all tool would be unrealistic. After you have taken a patient's comprehensive history using the questions in the Five-Dimension Assessment Model, revisit the patient's answers and discuss possible goals of care.

You may be thinking that using the Five-Dimension Assessment Model to help patients and families identify their goals of care will be more time-consuming than the method you're currently using. I would not disagree. This approach to setting goals requires an investment of time on the part of both provider and patient. The result is a plan of care designed to help the interdisciplinary/interprofessional team facilitate the achievement of each patient's unique goals for care. Patients and families are as unique as fingerprints: their goals of care should be unique as well.

HELPING PATIENTS AND FAMILIES ASSESS PROGRESS

In Chapter 4, we walked through the process of coordinating and facilitating the first meeting with a patient and family. The core principles for coordinating and facilitating family meetings remain the same throughout your work with that patient and family:

- The patient and the family (as identified by the patient) are the unit of care.
- Ask each patient, "Whom do you consider to be your family? Who are the people in your life who are sources of emotional support to you?" Then invite and facilitate the inclusion of those individuals in family meetings.
- Once a patient has identified the people they would like to have present at a family meeting, ask whether any of the individuals need an interpreter or have mobility, hearing, or visual impairments that you should be aware of, so you can ensure their access to and full participation in the family meeting. Enlist the help of the social worker or counselor on your interdisciplinary/interprofessional team to make the necessary arrangements to accommodate the needs of the patient and the family.

During every visit with a patient, as well as during each family meeting, revisit the patient's and family's goals of care and assess the progress toward expected outcomes. In palliative care and hospice care, goals should evolve over time to address changes in symptoms, psychosocial and spiritual needs, and caregiving concerns. If you are a physician, APRN, or RN, you're probably well versed in the practice of crafting new goals at each visit. Symptom management is a constantly moving target that requires both nimbleness and vigilance on the part of the clinician. If you are a social worker, counselor, or chaplain, though, you may notice from time to time that you are charting a fairly unchanged set of goals and expected outcomes over the course of weeks or months. If this happens, take a hard look at the way you are conducting assessments during your visits with the patient and family. As a patient's disease progresses, psychosocial and spiritual needs are likely to change — and goals of care should change too.

Interdisciplinary/interprofessional team meetings are the ideal forum in which to explore the evolving nature of the patient's and family's goals and expected outcomes. It is easy to fall into a routine, though, with the APRN or RN giving a report on the patient's condition and then other team members weighing in with their information. Instead of organizing team meetings around a discipline-by-discipline report on the patient and family, consider using the patient's and family's goals and expected outcomes as the framework for your team discussions. Another approach is to start the interdisciplinary/interprofessional team's discussion with a list of questions designed to keep the team focused on outcomes of care. You might also rotate which team member or discipline leads each meeting.

Chapter 4 discussed the Patient and Family Outcomes-Focused Inquiry for Developing Goals for Care, developed from the National Hospice and Palliative Care Organization's recommended outcomes for hospice and palliative care (Institute of Medicine and National Research Council 2003). Here, table 6.2 builds on that model, providing a framework for discussing patient and family goals for care during interdisciplinary/interprofessional team meetings. If you are part of a palliative care team that uses the case presentation model, consider incorporating some or all of these questions into your team discussions following presentations, as appropriate. To the right of each of the recommended outcomes listed in the table are questions you can ask yourself and other members of the team as you revisit and refine the patient's and family's goals of care. These questions constitute the core of what I call the Patient and Family Outcomes-Focused Inquiry for Interdisciplinary Teams.

If you work at one of the rare palliative care or hospice programs that still conducts physician-led, APRN-led, or RN-led interdisciplinary/interprofessional team meetings centered on the physician's or nurse's report, it may take some effort (and patience) to make the switch to structuring team discussions around the Patient and Family Outcomes-Oriented Inquiry framework. When your interdisciplinary/interprofessional team decides to give this approach a try, consider having one member of the team serve as the person who puts the questions before the team. Where team meetings have traditionally been run by the physician, APRN, or RN, try mixing things up a bit by asking the chaplain, social worker, or counselor to serve as the person posing the questions.

If you yourself are a physician, APRN, or RN, you may be feeling a twinge of discomfort at this suggestion. That's understandable given the central role that your discipline has probably played in interdisciplinary/interprofessional team meetings to this point, but it is important to remember that your role will not be diminished by having a member of another discipline pose questions to the team. On the contrary, you may find yourself contributing more substantively to the team discussions because you'll be answering the outcomes-oriented inquiry questions rather than spending your time and energy trying to facilitate the meeting.

Recommended outcomes[a]	Patient and family outcomes-focused inquiry: Questions to ask interdisciplinary team
Staff will prevent problems associated with coping, grieving, and existential results related to imminence of death [for patients near the end of life]	• What are we doing as a team to prevent problems associated with coping related to the imminence of death? • What, if any, are the patient's and family's goals and expected outcomes for coping with the imminence of death? • What are we doing as a team to prevent problems associated with grieving related to the imminence of death? • What, if any, are the patient's and family's goals and expected outcomes for grieving related to the imminence of death? • What are we doing as a team to prevent problems associated with existential issues related to the imminence of death? • What, if any, are the patient's and family's goals and expected outcomes for existential issues related to the imminence of death?
Staff will support the patient in achieving the optimal level of consciousness	• What are we doing as a team to support the patient in achieving the optimal level of consciousness? • How does the patient define the optimal level of consciousness? • How does the family define the optimal level of consciousness for the patient? • What, if any, are the patient's and family's goals and expected outcomes for achieving the optimal level of consciousness?
Staff will promote adaptive behaviors that are personally effective for the patient and family caregiver	• What are we doing as a team to promote adaptive behaviors that are personally effective for the patient? • What are the specific adaptive behaviors we are promoting? • What, if any, are the patient's and family's goals and expected outcomes related to these adaptive behaviors? • What are we doing to promote adaptive behaviors that are personally effective for the family caregiver? • What are the specific adaptive behaviors we are promoting? • What, if any, are the patient's and family's goals and expected outcomes related to these adaptive behaviors?
Staff will appropriately treat and prevent extension of disease and/or comorbidity	• What are we doing as a team to treat and prevent extension of the disease and/or comorbidity? • What, if any, are the patient's and family's goals and expected outcomes related to the treatment and prevention of extension of disease and/or comorbidity?
Staff will treat and prevent adverse effects of treatment	• What are we doing as a team to treat and prevent adverse effects of treatment? • What, if any, are the patient's and family's goals and expected outcomes related to the treatment and prevention of adverse effects of treatment?

Recommended outcomes[a]	Patient and family outcomes-focused inquiry: Questions to ask interdisciplinary team
Staff will treat and prevent distressing symptoms in concert with patient's wishes	• What are we doing as a team to treat and prevent distressing symptoms in concert with the patient's wishes? • What are the patient's wishes regarding the treatment and prevention of distressing symptoms? • What symptoms does the patient consider to be distressing? • What symptoms does the family consider to be distressing? • What, if any, are the patient's and family's goals and expected outcomes related to the treatment and prevention of distressing symptoms?
Staff will tailor treatments to patient's and family's functional capacity	• What are we doing as a team to tailor treatments to the patient's functional capacity? • What is the patient's functional capacity? • What are we doing as a team to tailor treatments to the family's functional capacity? • What is the family's functional capacity? • What, if any, are the patient's and family's goals and expected outcomes related to tailoring treatment to their functional capacity?
Staff will prevent crises from arising due to resource deficits	• What are we doing as a team to prevent crises from arising owing to resource deficits? • What are the existing resource deficits? What are the possible crises that may arise if these deficits are not addressed? • What, if any, are the patient's and family's goals and expected outcomes related to preventing crises arising owing to resource deficits?
Staff will respond appropriately to financial, legal, and environment problems that compromise care	• What are we doing as a team to respond appropriately to financial problems that compromise care? • What are the financial problems that could compromise care? • What, if any, are the patient's and family's goals and expected outcomes related to addressing financial problems that could compromise care? • What are we doing as a team to respond appropriately to legal problems that compromise care? • What are the legal problems that could compromise care? • What, if any, are the patient's and family's goals and expected outcomes related to addressing legal problems that could compromise care? • What are we doing as a team to respond appropriately to environmental problems that could compromise care? • What are the environmental problems that could compromise care? • What, if any, are the patient's and family's goals and expected outcomes related to addressing environmental problems that could compromise care?

continued

Recommended outcomes[a]	Patient and family outcomes-focused inquiry: Questions to ask interdisciplinary team
Staff will treat and prevent coping problems	• What are we doing as a team to treat and prevent the patient's coping problems? • What coping problems exist currently? • What coping problems are anticipated? • What, if any, are the patient's and family's goals and expected outcomes related to treating and preventing the patient's coping problems? • What are we doing as a team to treat and prevent the family's coping problems? • What coping problems exist currently for the family? • What coping problems are anticipated for the family? • What, if any, are the patient's and family's goals and expected outcomes related to treating and preventing the family's coping problems?
Staff will coach the patient and family through normal grieving	• What are we doing as a team to coach the patient through normal grieving? • What, if any, are the patient's and family's goals and expected outcomes related to coaching the patient through normal grieving? • What are we doing as a team to coach the family through normal grieving? • What, if any, are the patient's and family's goals and expected outcomes related to coaching the family through normal grieving?
Staff will assess and respond to anticipatory grief	• What are we doing as a team to assess and respond to the patient's anticipatory grief? • What, if any, are the patient's and family's goals and expected outcomes related to assessing and responding to the patient's anticipatory grief? • What are we doing as a team to assess and respond to the family's anticipatory grief? • What, if any, are the patient's and family's goals and expected outcomes related to assessing and responding to the family's anticipatory grief?
Staff will prevent unnecessary premature death	• What are we doing as a team to prevent unnecessary premature death? • How does the team define "unnecessary premature death"? • How does the patient define it? • How does the family define it? • What, if any, are the patient's and family's goals and expected outcomes related to preventing unnecessary premature death?

Recommended outcomes[a]	Patient and family outcomes-focused inquiry: Questions to ask interdisciplinary team
Staff will identify opportunities for family members' grief work	• What are we doing as a team to identify opportunities for family members' grief work? • What, if any, are the patient's and family's goals and expected outcomes related to identifying opportunities for family members' grief work?
Staff will assess the potential for complicated grief and respond appropriately	• What are we doing as a team to assess the potential for complicated grief? • What are we doing as a team to respond appropriately to complicated grief? • What, if any, are the patient's and family's goals for assessing and responding to complicated grief?
Staff will assist the family in integrating the memory of their loved one into their lives	• What are we doing as a team to assist the family in integrating the memory of their loved one into their lives? • What, if any, are the patient's and family's goals for integrating the memory of their loved one into their lives?

Source: Lunney et al. 2003.

[a] Text under "Recommended outcomes" © National Hospice and Palliative Care Organization and National Academy of Sciences. Reprinted with permission from the National Hospice and Palliative Care Organization and the National Academies Press.

ASSESSING AND ADDRESSING ENVIRONMENTAL AND SAFETY RISKS

Risk assessment is easiest when you can view the environment in person, so I will walk you through the process for conducting an in-home risk assessment before explaining how to carry out a risk assessment for a patient you are unable to visit at home.

The purpose of an **environmental and safety assessment** is twofold: to prevent falls and other accidents and to facilitate the continued independence of the patient. Before you begin an environmental and safety assessment, communicate to the patient, and to the family or others living in the home, if present, that you would like their permission to walk through their home in order to identify ways to help them make the home environment safer and easier for the patient to navigate. Make sure to let the patient and family know that you do this with all the patients you work with. Once the patient gives you permission to walk through the home, evaluate each room of the house and make notes on an assessment form.

If your palliative care service or hospice program has a standard assessment tool it prefers, use that tool to complete and document your assessment. Otherwise, I recommend using an assessment tool titled *Improving Independence in the Home Environment: Assessment and Intervention,* originally produced by the University of Buffalo's Center for Therapeutic Applications of Technology (Texas A&M AgriLife Extension n.d.). This assessment is short (just five pages long) and includes potential interventions for each problem identified. Once you have completed your environmental and safety assessment, circle your recommended interventions on the form and review them with the patient and family. To avoid overwhelming the patient and family, explain which of the interventions you and other members of the team will take care of for them, and when you will do so.

Consider proactively reaching out to your organization's volunteer coordinator to see if the coordinator would be open to recruiting volunteer handymen and handywomen to help implement the recommended safety interventions in patients' homes. Many of the interventions listed on the assessment form are simple tasks—for example, tacking down rugs, turning down the temperature on the water heater, and anchoring cords along the baseboard. Recruiting and training a cadre of volunteers to address the potential safety risks in patients' homes can give prospective volunteers a way to contribute their talents while also providing patients with a valuable service—one that can facilitate their continued independence.

When you see patients in a clinic and you are unable to assess their homes directly, you can use the University of Buffalo tool (or your program's preferred assessment tool) as a framework for discussing safety risks. For example, you can ask the patient and family whether they have unsafe features in the home—rolling beds, slippery floors, loose throw rugs, and so on—and discuss potential interventions. Alternatively, you can give patients a copy of the assessment form and encourage them to complete it at home and share the results with you at your next meeting. (This is the least desirable of the options, however, because it places the burden of assessment on the patients, and they may feel overwhelmed.)

Regardless of whether you conduct the environmental and safety assessment in person or through discussions with a patient, make sure to follow up with the patient to confirm that the safety risks you identified have been addressed. Assessing and documenting safety risks without later ensuring that those risks have been addressed is unwise; follow-through is essential.

A NOTE ABOUT OXYGEN USE IN THE HOME

When patients use oxygen in the home, you must pay particular attention to assessing, documenting, and addressing any safety risks you identify. LGBTQ individuals are more likely to be smokers than their cisgender and heterosexual counterparts, and this becomes an issue of particular concern when LGBTQ patients have oxygen tanks in the house. According to the Centers for Disease Control, the "smoking [rate] among lesbian, gay, and bisexual adults in the United States is much higher than among heterosexual/straight adults. Nearly 1 in 4 (23.9%) lesbian, gay, or bisexual adults smokes cigarettes[,] compared with roughly 1 in 6 (16.6%) heterosexual/straight adults" (CDC 2015).

Many patients, families, and even health care providers are unaware of the specific precautions that need to be taken to prevent a fire. Every hospice and palliative care provider knows that a patient should not smoke while connected to an oxygen tank, but did you know that it's not enough for the patient to disconnect the oxygen and go into another room in order to smoke safely? It is recommended that patients *wait*

Cynthia was a forty-eight-year-old widowed female with a primary diagnosis of chronic airway obstruction. Cynthia had wounds on her head and forehead from a burn sustained one week prior to hospice admission while staying at her sister's home. Cynthia and family reported that her oxygen concentrator was located too close to the furnace in her sister's house and the tube ignited, burning Cynthia's face. Cynthia was a smoker but denied that she was smoking when her oxygen caught fire. She was now living with her daughter Lisa. Also living in the home were Lisa's partner, Melinda, Melinda's mother, Norma, and Norma's son Joshua. Approximately one month after her hospice admission, there was an explosion and fire at Cynthia's daughter's home, which resulted in the deaths of Cynthia and Joshua. In addition to the deaths of their family members, Melinda and Lisa lost all of their personal items, even the clothes they had been wearing.

With the support of the Red Cross, a hotel room was found for Lisa and Melinda and clothing was provided, along with counseling support at their hotel room. The hospice's spiritual coordinator, Laurie, who visited Lisa and Melinda at the hotel, recalled that in addition to offering trauma counseling, she affirmed the relationship challenges and other social challenges Lisa and Melinda spoke of in relation to society and their sexual orientation. Laurie also recalled that she affirmed the support and strength they had provided for each other in their individual and shared challenges and how this could be seen as a strength in moving forward.

In this case, a very complicated and traumatic situation could have been made far worse if Melinda and Lisa's relationship was not accepted and honored by the hospice staff. Melinda was an active member of Cynthia's care team and managed her medications while also supporting Lisa, who was struggling emotionally with her own grief and health issues. Our hospice continued support of this couple following the fire tragedy at their home and provided additional counseling to them which both respected and recognized their close relationship as well as their losses.

—KUNGA NYIMA DROTOS, LMSW

ten minutes after discontinuing their oxygen and then *go outside to smoke*—and "even these steps cannot guarantee a person's safety. The safest course of action is to not smoke" (Massachusetts Executive Office of Public Safety n.d.).

Educate patients and families about the following precautions, which they should take to ensure their safety (Massachusetts Executive Office of Public Safety n.d.):

- Do not allow smoking in a home in which oxygen is being used. Smokers should go outside to smoke. If the patient is the smoker, he or she should wait ten minutes after turning off the oxygen before going outside and smoking. Keep electric razors, hair dryers, matches, candles, lighters, and gas stoves "at least 10 feet from the point where the oxygen comes out."
- Do not use aerosol sprays, petroleum jelly, lip balm, or oil-based lotions. These products can "spontaneously ignite when exposed to high oxygen concentrations."
- Put a sign on the front door of the home that reads "Oxygen in Use" so emergency responders (including firefighters) will know to take the proper precautions, should they need to enter the home.
- Make sure there are working smoke alarms throughout the house, and that they have fresh batteries.

- A plan of care should be "based on the identified and expressed preferences, values, goals, and needs of the patient and family and . . . developed with professional guidance and support for patient/family decision making" (National Consensus Project for Quality Palliative Care 2013).

- The patient's and family's goals for care and expected outcomes serve as the cornerstones for each plan of care.

- Expected outcomes—the outcomes of your interventions—should be measurable and time-limited: What will happen, and by when?

- Goals and expected outcomes will change over time. Work in collaboration with the patient, family, and other members of the interdisciplinary/interprofessional team to modify the plan of care as needed.

- It's easy to fall into a rut, charting the same goals of care over and over again for every patient, especially when you use an electronic health record that has a drop-down menu of often-cited goals. Resist the urge to take shortcuts when it comes to goals of care.

- During every visit with a patient, as well as during each family meeting, revisit the patient's and family's goals of care and assess progress toward expected outcomes.

- Interdisciplinary/interprofessional team meetings are the ideal forum in which to explore the evolving nature of the patient's and family's goals and expected outcomes.

- The Patient and Family Outcomes-Focused Inquiry for Interdisciplinary Teams provides a framework for discussing patient and family goals for care during team meetings. Consider incorporating some or all of these questions into your team discussions, as appropriate.

- The purpose of an environmental and safety assessment is twofold: to prevent falls and other accidents and to facilitate the continued independence of the patient.

- Regardless of whether you conduct the environmental and

safety assessment in person or through a discussion with the patient, make sure to follow up with the patient to make sure that risks have been addressed. Assessing and documenting safety risks without documenting that those risks have been addressed is unwise; follow-through is essential.

- If a patient is using oxygen in the home, pay particular attention to assessing, documenting, and addressing any safety risks. Because LGBTQ individuals are more likely to be smokers than their cisgender and heterosexual counterparts, this is an issue of particular concern when working with LGBTQ individuals who use oxygen in the home.
- It is not enough for patients to disconnect their oxygen and go into another room in order to smoke safely. Patients must *wait ten minutes after discontinuing their oxygen* and then *go outside to smoke*—and even these precautions won't guarantee their safety (Massachusetts Executive Office of Public Safety n.d.).
- Educate the patient and family about the precautions they should take to ensure their safety while using oxygen.

DISCUSSION QUESTIONS

1. What are the qualities of a well-crafted goal for care?
2. Imagine you are meeting with a patient to develop goals of care. Describe how you would help the patient and the patient's family formulate their goals of care and track progress toward expected outcomes.
3. Describe how an interdisciplinary/interprofessional team can stay focused on patient- and family-centered outcomes of care.
4. Imagine you are working with a new patient. How might you assess the patient's environmental and safety risks and provide suggestions for modifying the patient's environment to minimize safety risks?
5. Explain the precautions that patients, families, and staff need to take when oxygen is being used in the home.

Imagine that you have just been diagnosed with a life-threatening illness. Ask a colleague to write down five goals for your care without asking you any questions or talking to you about it. While they are writing down their goals for your care, write down your own five goals of care using the information in this chapter. Compare your goals with the goals written by your colleague. How has this activity changed your thoughts and feelings about the importance of patient-driven goals for care?

CHAPTER 7

ETHICAL AND LEGAL ISSUES

CHAPTER OBJECTIVES

1. Identify the ethical principles relevant to the provision of palliative care and hospice care.
2. Define and compare advance directive, advance care planning, living will, durable power of attorney for health care, will, POLST/MOLST, and do-not-resuscitate order.
3. List the ethical and legal issues that may affect LGBTQ individuals in particular.
4. Describe how you can help LGBTQ individuals and their families navigate the ethical and legal issues they may encounter.

Key Terms: advance care planning, advance directive, autonomy, beneficence, do-not-resuscitate order, durable power of attorney for health care, ethical principles, health care power of attorney, justice, living will, nonmaleficence, out-of-hospital/provider/physician/medical order for life-sustaining treatment (POLST/MOLST), will

Acquaviva, Kimberly
LGBTQ-Inclusive Hospice and Palliative Care
dx.doi.org/10.17312/harringtonparkpress/2017.03lgbtqihpc.007
© 2017 by Kimberly Acquaviva

Palliative-care and hospice professionals have a duty to the patients and families they work with—of all sexual orientations, gender identities, and gender expressions—to adhere to a core set of ethical principles in carrying out their work. These ethical principles compel them to honor the autonomy of the people they serve. In health care, autonomy is "protected" through the **advance care planning** process. Surgeon and author Atul Gawande writes of the true meaning of autonomy in *Being Mortal*: "He moved his line in the sand. This is what it means to have autonomy—you may not control life's circumstances, but getting to be the author of your life means getting to control what you do with them" (Gawande 2014). This chapter provides an overview of the ethical principles that guide practice, the elements of advance care planning, and the legal issues that may affect LGBTQ individuals in particular as they navigate serious and life-threatening illness and seek to remain the authors of their own lives.

None of the following information is intended to constitute legal advice, nor is it my intent to encourage you to provide legal advice to your patients and their families. The information in this chapter is designed to make you aware of some of the ethical and legal issues that LGBTQ individuals and their families may encounter so that you can provide support and guidance within the scope of your professional discipline. For a deeper dive into ethics as they relate to health care delivery, I highly recommend Beauchamp and Childress's *Principles of Biomedical Ethics* (2013).

ETHICAL PRINCIPLES AND THEIR RELEVANCE TO CARE DELIVERY

Your work as a hospice or palliative care professional should be shaped by the four principles that define your ethical duties to the patients and families you serve (Beauchamp and Childress 2013):

- **Autonomy:** Honor the right of patients and families to make their own decisions.
- **Beneficence:** Help patients and families benfit (in ways defined by each patient and family).
- **Nonmaleficence:** Do no harm to patients or their families.
- **Justice:** Be fair and treat all patients and families equitably.

It can be challenging to uphold all four ethical principles simultaneously. One might even argue that it's impossible to uphold all four principles in equal measure at all times. Imagine you are working with a man who has stage IV lung cancer, brain metastases, and mild cognitive impairment. The patient tells you during your first meeting that, given his limited life expectancy, he plans to continue smoking. The patient has been experiencing severe dyspnea for the past few weeks and uses oxygen at home. You have explained the risks associated with smoking while on oxygen, but the patient insists that he wants to continue to smoke until he dies. The patient assures you he will smoke only outside the home, and only after waiting for ten minutes after he has discontinued his oxygen use. You convey to the patient and his family caregiver that even those precautions will not eliminate the risk of fire, but the patient is unmoved.

In this scenario, there is a clear conflict between following the principles of autonomy and beneficence. Despite your best efforts to convince the patient of the dangers of smoking while on oxygen, the patient is asserting his right to make an autonomous choice to continue to smoke. The patient's cognitive impairment complicates things, however: Can a patient make an autonomous choice under a condition of mild cognitive impairment? Your duty of beneficence compels you to protect the patient and his family from harm. Further complicating things is the fact that your duty of nonmaleficence prevents you from discontinuing the patient's oxygen because that would cause the patient to suffer. How can you reconcile these conflicting principles in a way that meets the needs of the patient while also meeting your need to uphold the ethical principles?

Unless a patient lacks the capacity for decision making, upholding the principle of autonomy should be your primary goal, followed closely by the other three ethical principles. The patient in the scenario described has mild cognitive impairment, but in the opinion of the physician and the rest of the care team, he still has the capacity to make an autonomous decision to continue to smoke. The patient has indicated a willingness to take certain precautions to reduce the risk of fire in the home. In striving to uphold the principle of beneficence, you might meet with the patient and family caregiver together to review the safety concerns and recommended precautions, so that everyone is on the same page regarding the risks and precautions being taken in the home. The safety precautions are not simply for the benefit of the patient and family: the principle of beneficence extends to the surrounding community as well. Home oxygen fires result in injuries, death, and loss of property, all of which are "harms" you should seek to prevent.

ADVANCE CARE PLANNING

When a patient is facing a serious or life-limiting illness, they may be fearful of the uncertain future that lies ahead. Although you can't predict everything the patient is going to experience in the weeks, months, or years to come, you can increase the patient's feeling of control and reduce fear of the unknown by helping with advance care planning. Advance care planning is an overarching term used to describe the process of identifying, discussing, and executing plans for future health care decisions. The Institute of Medicine's report *Dying in America* notes the importance of advance care planning, asserting that "fundamental to the advance care planning process is clear empathetic communication between clinicians and patients, which can lead to shared decision-making" (Institute of Medicine 2015). While experts encourage all

Ben and Jeff were a couple who had been together for twenty years. Ben was an art collector and Jeff was a businessman. They lived in a condominium that they had renovated together. Ben was estranged from his family. Ben developed heart failure. He continued active treatment. However, one day he went into heart failure and was admitted to the medical intensive care unit. Jeff visited regularly. Ben's condition declined suddenly and he became unconscious.

Unfortunately, Ben and Jeff had never completed surrogate decision-maker paperwork. Therefore, Jeff was not legally able to make decisions. Contact was made with Ben's family. They came to the intensive care unit to visit Ben once. The health care team held a family meeting to discuss comfort measures. Ben's family stated that they had not agreed with Ben's "lifestyle" and they wanted him to suffer. The team stated that, ethically, they needed to treat his heart failure. Again Ben's family stated that they believed allowing him to suffer would help him atone for his sins. The health care team explained that their code of ethics mandated appropriate management of pain and symptoms. The family forbade Jeff to visit, stating he had made Ben sin. The team explained that Jeff was Ben's family and had been a support person over the course of his disease. Moreover, Ben had stated he wanted Jeff there.

The family left and never returned, even when Ben died. The team allowed Jeff to see Ben to say good-bye and offered support.

—CONSTANCE DAHLIN, ANP-BC, ACHPN

adults to engage in advance care planning conversations, when patients have a serious or life-limiting illness the planning process can help them clarify and express their goals of care to family and care providers.

YOUR ROLE IN ADVANCE CARE PLANNING

As a palliative care or hospice professional, your role (in collaboration with other members of the interdisciplinary/ interprofessional team) in the advance care planning process consists of four core tasks: (1) identifying the patient's current understanding of the illness; (2) providing the patient with information about treatment options, benefits, and burdens; (3) facilitating discussions between the patient and family regarding the patient's treatment options, preferences, and decisions; and (4) assisting the patient in documenting preferences and decisions in writing. I have intentionally kept the first two tasks focused on the patient (as opposed to both the patient and family) because each patient should be given the opportunity to explore and express treatment options, preferences, and decisions with their health care provider without the presence or influence of family members or other caregivers. Since clinicians gained the ability in 2016 to bill for advance care planning under Medicare, palliative care providers are well positioned to partner with social workers, counselors, and other members of the team in delivering this valuable service to the patients and families they serve.

While the patient and family are considered to be the unit of care in hospice and palliative care, there is substantial value in providing patients with a safe space in which to explore and express their own questions, concerns, and preferences before the patient's family is brought into the conversation. A patient may want to discontinue curative treatment or talk with you about forgoing resuscitation, but they may be reluctant to express that desire in front of their spouse, partner, adult child, or other family member. Whenever possible, talk with the patient one on one. Once you have a clear sense of the patient's wishes, you can facilitate a discussion between the patient and family toward the dual goal of supporting the patient's decisions and assisting the family in understanding and supporting the patient's wishes. The third task, facilitating patient-family discussions, depends on family dynamics and the patient's preferences.

Although there are four core tasks in the advance care planning process, the process is more iterative than linear. Advance care planning is intended to be an ongoing process, supporting patient-identified goals and decisions. It is not uncommon, for example, for patients who were initially in favor of resuscitation to change their mind as their condition worsens. Likewise, patients who were strongly opposed to receiving artificial nutrition or hydration when they were first diagnosed may change their mind if there is a major life event (e.g., birth of a grandchild, wedding, graduation) they are trying to live long enough to witness. As conditions and circumstances change, patients' wishes and decisions may evolve, and often do. (*Note:* When patients state in their advance directive that they want to receive artificial nutrition and hydration and a hospice program is unwilling or unable to provide that service, it would be unethical for that hospice to admit them.)

Palliative and hospice care professionals weave the first two tasks in the process into regular goals-of-care discussions, to affirm the patient's understanding of the illness and provide treatment options. If a patient's goals of care or treatment choices change, then additional patient and family discussions may be needed.

ADVANCE CARE PLANNING DOCUMENTS

As a palliative care or hospice professional, you may already be familiar with the different kinds of documents involved in the advance care planning process. Following is a quick refresher for professionals who are less familiar with advance care documents.

The term **advance directive** encompasses two separate and distinct legal documents: the health care power of attorney and the living will (National Hospice and Palliative Care Organization 2016). State regulations guide the execution and implementation of advance directives, with some states detailing the specific content and format of each document. Some states—California is one—use the term *advance health care directive* to describe a document that combines a health care power of attorney and a living will.

A **health care power of attorney** (also called a **durable power of attorney for health care**) specifies the individual—sometimes referred to as the health care agent, **health care proxy**, or health care surrogate—authorized by the patient to make health care decisions in the event that the patient is no longer capable of communicating treatment decisions to health care providers. The power of attorney (POA) document typically names a primary decision maker and also a "backup" decision maker who is authorized to make decisions in the event the primary person is unable to fulfill that role. The decision maker can be the person's spouse, adult child, another relative, or a close friend. State laws govern the restrictions regarding who can serve as the POA, including prohibitions against health care providers or paid caregivers serving in that role.

An individual appointed to serve as a health care POA is authorized to make medical decisions only in the event the patient is temporarily or permanently incapacitated owing to an illness or accident. Unlike a legal or financial power of attorney, the health care POA authorizes that individual to make only medical decisions on the patient's behalf. Similarly, a person holding legal or financial power of attorney is authorized to make only legal or financial decisions and does not have the authority to make medical decisions for a patient.

When a patient does not have a documented health care POA, state law specifies the person authorized to make medical decisions for the patient—the default decision maker.

Each state delineates a list of default surrogate decision makers, in hierarchical order, so that health care providers in that state can determine who is authorized to make decisions. (This person is sometimes referred to as the "next of kin.") Typically the first default decision maker is the person's legally recognized spouse. In the absence of a spouse, the next person listed varies depending on state statutes but is typically a person related to the patient (Williamson, Lesandrini, and Kamdar 2016; Wynn 2014).

Having a health care POA is extremely important for unmarried LGBTQ individuals, especially for those who are estranged from one or more family members. Unmarried life partners can be excluded from the decision-making process, or even prevented from seeing the patient, at the discretion of the default decision maker. Therefore the ethical principles of autonomy and beneficence dictate that health care providers must educate the patient and family of choice about the importance of executing a health care power of attorney.

A **living will** enables individuals to codify in writing the specific treatments they do or do not want to receive in the event they become unable to communicate their wishes. Although a written living will is the most commonly encountered form, the Institute of Medicine has a broader definition: "A written or video statement about the kind of medical care a person does or does not want under certain specific conditions if no longer able to express those wishes" (Institute of Medicine 2015). The types of treatments outlined in a living will may include but are not limited to: cardiopulmonary resuscitation (CPR), artificial nutrition or hydration, antibiotics, surgery, and use of a ventilator.

Patients and families should be able to obtain forms for a living will from your palliative care or hospice program, and they can also obtain them from their local area agency on aging (see, e.g., www.eldercare.gov), their state health department, from the organization Aging with Dignity (https://www.agingwithdignity.org/five-wishes), and from CaringInfo, a program of the National Hospice and Palliative Care Organization (www.caringinfo.org). The Conversation Project (www.theconversationproject.org) offers free, downloadable "starter kits" that can be helpful for patients and families before they begin the process of completing a living will.

Many states allow patients to include supplementary instructions about a particular treatment that they wish to allow only for a specified period of time. For example, a patient may opt to be placed on a ventilator for a short period of time in the event of an acute crisis so long as the ventilator is discontinued if the patient cannot survive without mechanical ventilation. Or they may specifically request palliative or hospice care in the living will so their health care providers will make a referral to palliative or hospice care.

If a patient has a living will and a health care power of attorney, these must be documented in the medical record. In the absence of a living will, the health care providers must rely on the individual designated in the health care power of attorney or a default decision maker to make decisions if the patient is incapacitated. If decision makers are unavailable, then health care professionals are required to provide life-sustaining treatments. Without a health care power of attorney and living will, a patient may receive treatment that is unwanted and that can potentially lead to prolonged suffering. For example, patients with dementia who are given artificial nutrition and hydration while they are actively dying may suffer discomfort as the body works to process the nutrients when its systems are shutting down.

A do-not-resuscitate (DNR) order, sometimes called a *do-not-attempt-resuscitation (DNAR) order* or *allow-natural-death (AND) order,* is a signed medical order that instructs care providers not to perform cardiopulmonary resuscitation (CPR) if the patient stops breathing or the patient's heart stops beating. While patients can request a DNR either verbally or in their living will, a health care practitioner must sign the order and place it in the patient's medical record. Congruent with the principle of autonomy, the health care practitioner should contact the patient or decision maker to confirm that a DNR is desired before writing the order.

An **out-of-hospital/provider/physician/medical order for life-sustaining treatment (POLST/MOLST)** varies from state to state in name, format, and powers, but in general it "provides medical orders for *current treatment*" (emphasis added) for "persons with serious illness" (National POLST Paradigm 2015). The POLST form "complements the Advance Directive and is not intended to replace it. An Advance Directive is necessary to appoint a legal health care representative and provide instructions for *future* life-sustaining treatments" (ibid.).

Patients and families are sometimes confused about the difference between a health care power of attorney and a legal or financial power of attorney. Again, the individual designated by a patient to serve as their health care power of attorney is authorized to make only health care decisions— decisions a person given legal or financial power of attorney would be unable to make. If a patient tells you they have completed a health care power of attorney, ask for a copy of it for the patient's chart or medical record and make sure that team members from all shifts are aware of the designated decision maker. If the document the patient gives you is actually a legal or financial power of attorney, return it and offer to walk the patient through completing a health care power of attorney.

Patients and families also get confused about the difference between a **living will** and a **will** (or last will and testament. A living will is a document expressing a patient's health care treatment preferences. In contrast, a last will and testament is a financial document that allows patients to plan who receives their financial assets and property (National Hospice and Palliative Care Organization 2016).

As with a health care power of attorney, if a patient says they have a living will, ask to make a copy of it for the chart or medical record. If the document the patient gives you is actually a will, give it back and ask if you can help by walking the patient through the process of completing a living will.

HELPING LGBTQ PATIENTS NAVIGATE LEGAL ISSUES

Within the context of a serious or life-limiting illness, LGBTQ individuals and their families may encounter difficulty with legal issues in three overarching areas: health care decision making, disposition of remains, and property ownership. These issues are not unique to LGBTQ individuals, and you should be aware of them as you begin working with any new patient and family. LGBTQ individuals who want to create legal documents without hiring an attorney can often do so online by using LGBTQ-friendly sites such as http://www.legalout.com. However, individuals and families who have complex legal and/or financial issues and concerns should be encouraged to consult with an attorney for guidance.

HEALTH CARE DECISION MAKING

In the absence of a properly executed advance directive such as a health care power of attorney, the right to make decisions for a patient who is incapable of making decisions autonomously generally falls to a legal spouse and then to other relatives, although the default hierarchy varies from state to state. Patients may be in a long-term relationship that they consider to be a marriage, but in the absence of a marriage certificate, that relationship may not be legally recognized. This is true whether the relationship is between two men, two women, or a man and a woman.

Never assume that words like *married, spouse, husband,* and *wife* mean that a relationship has been formalized legally. When patients use terms like these to refer to a person who is significant to them, follow up, in a way that is both non-judgmental and affirming, to ascertain whether the relationship has been formalized legally. For example, you might say something like this to a patient: "I want to make sure you have the documents you need to protect your right to involve [name of individual] in your care. Sometimes couples choose to formalize their relationship through a legally recognized process such as a marriage or domestic partnership. If you have not done that, don't worry—there are easy ways I can help you put things in writing if you choose to, so that [name of individual] or someone else can act on your behalf if need be." Let the patient know you are asking about the relationship not out of curiosity but to help you better understand who the patient's default decision maker will be if there is no health care power of attorney on file.

DISPOSITION OF REMAINS

A patient's death can clearly be very upsetting to caregivers, other family members, and friends. Conflict over the patient's remains can compound the distress experienced by all those involved. A *funeral directive* or *disposition-of-remains directive* is a tool that can ensure that the wishes of the patient are honored after death. The potential consequences of forgoing a funeral directive for LGBTQ individuals can be substantial:

> If [patients do] not record [their] wishes in a legal document, the law defaults to the person or people [their] state defines as [their] "next of kin" to make these decisions for [them]—usually a blood relative. If [patients have] a spouse or registered domestic partner legally recognized in [their] state or the state where the death occurs, that person probably will stand ahead of [the patient's] blood relatives. [Patients will] want to establish who will be in charge, and also make [their] wishes about the arrangements clear in writing so as to prevent arguments. If [patients do] not leave binding written instructions, someone [they] haven't chosen could decide everything from whether [their] organs will be donated to whether [they] will be buried or cremated, from what [their] memorial service will be to the clothing [they] will be buried in, from the

language [on their] headstone to how [their] gender identity is listed in an obituary. (Lambda Legal 2014)

When working with transgender patients, it is vitally important that you encourage them to put their wishes in writing in the form of a funeral directive. Although this document may seem redundant if disposition of remains is covered in a durable power of attorney, will, or other legal document, legal complexities are such that redundancy may be wise in order to allay patients' concerns about how they will be dressed, referred to, and honored after their death. Patients do not need to hire a lawyer to draw up a funeral directive. A funeral directive can be written by the patient, then signed and dated in the presence of a notary public (Lambda Legal 2014).

PROPERTY OWNERSHIP

The third area in which LGBTQ individuals and their families may encounter legal issues is property ownership. If a patient shares a home with a partner or friend who is not their legal spouse, beneficiary, or joint tenant, upon the death of the patient there is nothing to protect the partner or friend from being put out on the street by the patient's biological family. A less extreme outcome, but still distressing to a grieving partner or friend, could be the removal of jewelry, mementos, artwork, furniture, photo albums, computers, and other personal property from the home by members of the patient's biological family. Unfortunately, a "same-sex partner or a friend not named as a beneficiary in a Will, or as a joint tenant on a property deed or in trust, could find all the property belonging to the deceased going to the deceased's children, parents, siblings or other biological family members against the deceased's intention" (Wenzel 2015). When you are working with a lesbian, gay, bisexual, transgender, gender-nonconforming, queer, and/or questioning patient, be aware of the possibility that the patient and caregiver may be anxious

- Who should have authority over your remains?
- Do you wish to be an organ donor? If so, have you indicated that on your driver's license? In your health care proxy and/or funeral directive? Do you wish to make any restrictions on the organs available for donation, and are those wishes documented?
- Who should have authority to make funeral-related decisions?
- Do you have wishes for a particular funeral home and how much money should be spent? Do you have particular wishes for a casket?
- Do you want a wake or "viewing"? If so, do you have preferences as to whether your casket is open or closed, or what clothing and makeup should be used?
- Do you want cremation?
- Do you want burial, regardless of whether or not you are cremated?
- Do you have strong feelings about what should happen at your memorial service? Do you want your service to invoke a religious tradition?
- Do you have wishes about a particular cemetery, headstone, and maintenance of the plot, or about some alternative way that you wish to be remembered in the future?
- If you have a spouse or partner, how do you want that person described in your obituary? How would you like your gender identity described and what name and pronouns should be used? Do you have any other specific wishes for how you and your life are described?

From Lambda Legal 2014. Reprinted with permission. © 2014 Lambda Legal.

The hospice where I work admitted Jim, an elderly married man with a primary diagnosis of a stroke. Jim lived at an independent living center and was supported by his spouse, Bob. Jim and Bob had been together for fifty-seven years but had just been married the week before Jim was admitted to hospice. Their marriage was made possible by the Supreme Court decision a few weeks earlier in support of same sex marriages. Bob reported that Jim had grown up in Battle Creek, and they met when Jim's car broke down at a rest area off the highway and Bob gave him a ride home.

Bob reported that getting married after fifty-seven years together was purely a business decision to protect their assets from family members who might not respect their relationship, or their wills. Specifically, Bob stated that there were several lawyers in the family who might try to contest Jim's will. Jim had a sister in a city a few hours away, but the couple had no local family support. Jim was unable to provide any personal information to hospice staff, owing to the effects of his stroke. Bob stated that he and his spouse used to enjoy having dinner with friends and throwing large parties several times a year. Since Jim's decline and the couple's relocation to an assisted living facility, Bob was mainly supported by phone contact with friends who lived out of town and by some local friends at the facility. Jim and Bob were at higher risk for bereavement issues because they had limited family support as well as stress related to concerns that family members would contest Jim's dying wishes. Their right to marry was a contested issue, and the media at the time were saturated with stories and opinions both in support of and against same-sex marriage. Bob and Jim lived in a small, conservative community where there were no bereavement support groups for same-sex couples.

—KUNGA NYIMA DROTOS, LMSW

about something like this happening to them. Anticipatory grief can be complicated by worries about impending conflicts over property, so connect the patient and caregiver with the resources they need to put their legal affairs in order.

WHO NEEDS TO KNOW? ENSURING CONFIDENTIALITY

During the care planning and coordination process, you will probably be communicating with a variety of professionals and laypeople outside your interdisciplinary/interprofessional team. In the course of providing and coordinating care, you might interact with the patient's primary care provider, spiritual advisor, counselor or therapist, family members, friends, and neighbors, among others. The Health Insurance Portability and Accountability Act (known as HIPAA) prohibits you from disclosing a patient's "protected health information" (including sexual orientation, sex anatomy, and gender identity) without the patient's permission, except in certain situations outlined in the law. In general, you should not share information about a patient's sex anatomy, gender identity, and sexual orientation outside the interdisciplinary/interprofessional team without the patient's permission, even if HIPAA allows such disclosures without the patient's consent.

When patients' sex anatomy and gender identity do not match, your use of their preferred gender pronouns may inadvertently "out" them to friends and family. When patients tell you which gender pronouns they prefer, ask them if there is anyone with whom you should avoid using those pronouns. For example, a patient who was assigned the female sex at birth and now identifies as male may not want to be referred to as "he" or "him" in front of his parents. Do not assume this is the case, however: a transgender patient's family of origin may be completely accepting of the patient's gender identity.

Information about sex anatomy should be shared only with individuals who have a clinical need to know that information. For example, a home health aide making a home visit to assist a patient with bathing should be informed if the patient's sex anatomy and gender identity do not align. Ideally, home health aides should be able to deliver high-quality patient care to transgender patients without getting a heads-up before their interaction with the patient, but the reality is that not all home health aides have had the benefit of education regarding the care of transgender patients. Transgender patients should never be made to feel as though they are their care provider's "teachable moment," nor should transgender patients be subjected to care from a provider who acts shocked or flummoxed by the appearance of a patient's genitals. (This principle extends to the care of *all* patients in palliative care and hospice care.)

It is difficult to imagine a situation in which it would be clinically relevant to share information about a patient's sexual orientation with individuals outside the interdisciplinary/interprofessional team. More likely to occur are inadvertent disclosures resulting from making reference to a patient's partner. If the patient self-identifies as lesbian, gay, or bisexual and is currently with a partner, ask if there is anyone with whom you should avoid making reference to that partner. Regardless of whether they are currently with a partner, if patients self-identify as lesbian, gay, or bisexual, ask them if there are any significant individuals in their life who are unaware of their sexual orientation. It's important for patients to be able to trust that you will maintain **confidentiality** and prevent information about their sexual orientation from being disclosed inappropriately.

When in doubt about whether a particular disclosure is both necessary and appropriate, ask yourself the following questions:

- Can the patient receive the best care possible *without* this information being disclosed?
- If I do not disclose this information to a provider, could the patient be subjected to insensitive or poor-quality

care by that provider? If so, is there a way I can prevent the patient from being subjected to insensitive or poor-quality care *without* disclosing the information?

- Am I disclosing this information to meet my own needs or the needs of the patient?
- Does the patient want this information to be disclosed? How do I know that?

KEY POINTS TO REMEMBER

- Your duty to the patients and families you work with—of all sexual orientations, gender identities, and gender expressions—is to adhere to a core set of ethical principles in carrying out your work. These ethical principles compel you to honor the autonomy of the people you serve. In health care, autonomy should be supported and protected through the advance care planning process.
- As a hospice or palliative care professional, your work should be shaped by the four principles that define your ethical duties to the patients and families you serve: autonomy, beneficence, nonmaleficence, and justice.
- Although you can't predict everything a patient is going to experience in the weeks, months, or years to come, you can increase patients' sense of control and reduce their fear of the unknown by helping them with advance care planning.
- Advance care planning is intended to be an ongoing process, supporting patient-identified goals and decisions. As patients' conditions and circumstances change, their wishes and decisions may also evolve, and often do.
- Appointing a health care POA is extremely important for unmarried LGBTQ individuals, especially those who are estranged from one or more family members. The ethical principles of autonomy and beneficence dictate that health care providers must educate the patient and family of choice about the importance of executing a health care power of attorney.

- Within the context of a serious or life-limiting illness, LGBTQ individuals and their families may encounter difficulty with legal issues in three overarching areas: health care decision making, disposition of remains, and property ownership. These issues are not unique to LGBTQ individuals and their families, and you should be aware of these issues as you begin working with any new patient and family.

- HIPAA prohibits you from disclosing a patient's "protected health information" (including sexual orientation, sex anatomy, and gender identity) without the patient's permission, except in certain situations outlined in the law. In general, you should not share information about a patient's sex anatomy, gender identity, and sexual orientation outside the interdisciplinary/interprofessional team without the patient's permission, even if HIPAA allows such disclosures without the patient's consent.

- When patients' sex anatomy and gender identity do not match, your use of their preferred gender pronouns may inadvertently "out" them to friends and family. When patients tell you their preferred gender pronouns, ask them if there is anyone with whom you should avoid using those pronouns.

- Information about sex anatomy should be shared only with individuals who have a clinical need to know that information.

DISCUSSION QUESTIONS

1. What are the ethical principles relevant to the provision of palliative care and hospice care? Which of these ethical principles do you think are the most important? Which do you think are the most difficult to uphold?

2. Advance directive documents can be confusing even to experienced health care professionals—it's not surprising that professionals new to the field might be confused. Imagine that you are working with a recent graduate in

your discipline who has asked you to explain the following concepts: advance directive, advance care planning, living will, durable power of attorney for health care, POLST/MOLST, and DNR order. What would you say?

3. What are some of the ethical and legal issues that may affect LGBTQ individuals in particular in palliative and hospice care?

4. Describe how you would help an LGBTQ patient and family navigate the ethical and legal issues that they might encounter when facing a serious or life-threatening illness.

5. When is disclosing a patient's "protected health information" (including sexual orientation, sex anatomy, and gender identity) permitted? How might the use of gendered pronouns constitute a breach of HIPAA?

CHAPTER ACTIVITY

Complete a living will and a durable power of attorney for health care using free resources available on the Internet. Make sure the forms you use are valid in the state in which you live. Share the documents with your primary health care provider as well as with at least one member of your family. After you have completed the documents, reflect on what the process was like for you. Was it easier or harder than you had anticipated? How do you think your choices and preferences might change over the course of your lifetime? How often do you think you might revisit (and if necessary revise) these documents?

CHAPTER 8

PATIENT AND FAMILY EDUCATION AND ADVOCACY

CHAPTER OBJECTIVES

1. Explain how to assess knowledge of patient care and teach patient-care skills.
2. Explain how to assess knowledge and teach patients and caregivers about end-stage disease progression.
3. Explain how to assess knowledge and teach patients and caregivers about pain and symptom management.
4. Explain how to assess knowledge and teach patients and caregivers about medication management.
5. Explain how to assess knowledge and teach patients and caregivers about disposal of supplies.
6. Explain how to assess knowledge and teach patients and caregivers about the signs and symptoms of imminent death.

Key Terms: disposal of supplies, end-stage disease progression, medication management, medication reconciliation, pain and symptom management, patient-care skills, signs and symptoms of imminent death

Acquaviva, Kimberly
LGBTQ-Inclusive Hospice and Palliative Care
dx.doi.org/10.17312/harringtonparkpress/2017.03lgbtqihpc.008
© 2017 by Kimberly Acquaviva

Patient and family education is an essential part of delivering quality care (Institute of Medicine 2013). Education is an integral part of the work that advanced practice registered nurses, physicians, registered nurses, chaplains, social workers, and counselors do with patients and families. This chapter provides palliative care and hospice professionals with specific, actionable strategies for teaching patients and families (including but not limited to those who are LGBTQ) about patient care, end-stage disease progression, **pain and symptom management**, medication management, the **disposal of supplies**, and **signs and symptoms of imminent death**.

HOW TO ASSESS PRIOR KNOWLEDGE AND TEACH PATIENT-CARE SKILLS

If you are a physician, advanced practice registered nurse, or registered nurse and you're preparing to teach **patient-care skills** to a patient and a family caregiver, a good place to start is with the patient's answers to the questions about activities of daily living in Dimension 3 of the Five-Dimension Assessment Model, discussed in Chapter 4. The patient's answers to those questions will give you much of the information you need to provide focused education to the patient; the missing piece will be understanding the caregiver's knowledge and needs. Before you ask questions to assess the caregiver's knowledge about patient care, let the caregiver know that your questions are designed to help you provide better support, not to see whether the caregiver is doing a "good" or "bad" job caring for the patient.

In assessing a caregiver's knowledge of and need for particular patient-care skills, you should ask four key questions. The caregiver's answers will give you the information you need to teach the patient-care skills in question. Each question aligns with a teaching task, described in greater depth in table 8.1.

TABLE 8.1 ASSESSING AND TEACHING PATIENT-CARE SKILLS

Questions for assessing patient and caregiver knowledge and needs	Addressing knowledge and needs when teaching patient-care skills
BATHING	
Walk me through how you [help patient] bathe. What tasks are the most difficult for you in terms of bathing [patient]? What challenges or problems have you encountered in bathing [patient]? What questions or concerns do you have regarding bathing [patient]?	Offer concrete praise to the patient and caregiver regarding at least one aspect of the process they've been using for bathing. Provide focused education for any bathing tasks that the patient or caregiver has been performing incorrectly (based on their description of the bathing process). Provide focused education for each bathing task the patient or caregiver identifies as having been difficult. Provide specific strategies for overcoming or addressing the challenges the patient or caregiver has encountered in the bathing process. Answer the patient's and caregiver's questions and address their concerns regarding bathing.
GETTING DRESSED	
Walk me through how you [help patient] get dressed. What tasks are the most difficult for you in terms of dressing [patient]? What challenges or problems have you encountered in dressing [patient]? What questions or concerns do you have regarding dressing [patient]?	Offer concrete praise to the patient and caregiver regarding at least one aspect of the dressing process they've been using. Provide focused education for any dressing tasks that the patient or caregiver has been performing incorrectly (based on their description of the process). Provide focused education for each dressing task the patient or caregiver identifies as having been difficult. Provide specific strategies for overcoming or addressing the challenges the patient or caregiver has encountered when dressing the patient. Answer the patient's and caregiver's questions and address their concerns regarding dressing the patient.
MEALS AND EATING	
Walk me through how you [help patient] prepare meals and eat. What tasks are the most difficult for you in terms of preparing meals and eating [feeding patient]?	Offer concrete praise to the patient and caregiver regarding at least one aspect of the process of the meal preparation and feeding process they've been using. Provide focused education for any meal prep and feeding tasks that the patient or caregiver has been performing incorrectly (based on their description of the process). Provide focused education for each meal prep and feeding task the patient or caregiver identifies as having been difficult.

Questions for assessing patient and caregiver knowledge and needs	Addressing knowledge and needs when teaching patient-care skills
What challenges or problems have you encountered preparing meals and eating [feeding patient]? What questions or concerns do you have regarding preparing meals and eating [feeding patient]?	Provide focused education for each meal prep and feeding task the patient or caregiver identifies as having been difficult. Provide specific strategies for overcoming or addressing the challenges the patient or caregiver has encountered when preparing meals for and feeding the patient. Answer the patient's and caregiver's questions and address their concerns regarding preparing meals for and feeding the patient

GETTING OUT OF BED

Walk me through how you [help patient] get out of bed. What tasks are the most difficult for you in terms of getting [patient] out of bed? What challenges or problems have you encountered getting [patient] out of bed? What questions or concerns do you have regarding getting [patient] out of bed?	Offer concrete praise to the patient and caregiver regarding at least one aspect of the process they've been using to get the patient out of bed. Provide focused education for any tasks that the patient or caregiver has been performing incorrectly (based on their description of the process). Provide focused education for each task the patient or caregiver identifies as having been difficult in terms of getting the patient out of bed. Provide specific strategies for overcoming or addressing the challenges the patient or caregiver has encountered when getting the patient out of bed. Answer the patient's and caregiver's questions and address their concerns regarding getting the patient out of bed.

MOVING FROM BED TO CHAIR

Walk me through how you [help patient] move from the bed to the chair. What tasks are the most difficult for you in terms of moving [patient] from the bed to the chair? What challenges or problems have you encountered moving [patient] from the bed to the chair? What questions or concerns do you have regarding moving [patient] from the bed to the chair?	Offer concrete praise to the patient and caregiver regarding at least one aspect of the process they've been using to move the patient from the bed to the chair. Provide focused education for any tasks that the patient or caregiver has been performing incorrectly (based on their description of the process). Provide focused education for each task the patient or caregiver identifies as having been difficult in terms of moving the patient from the bed to the chair. Provide specific strategies for overcoming or addressing the challenges the patient or caregiver has encountered when moving the patient from the bed to the chair. Answer the patient's and caregiver's questions and address their concerns regarding moving the patient from the bed to the chair.

continued

Questions for assessing patient and caregiver knowledge and needs	Addressing knowledge and needs when teaching patient-care skills

MOVING FROM CHAIR TO BATHROOM

Walk me through how you [help patient] move from the chair to the bathroom.	Offer concrete praise to the patient and caregiver regarding at least one aspect of the process they've been using to move the patient from the chair to the bathroom.
What tasks are the most difficult for you in terms of moving [patient] from the chair to the bathroom?	Provide focused education for any tasks that the patient or caregiver has been performing incorrectly (based on their description of the process).
What challenges or problems have you encountered moving [patient] from the chair to the bathroom?	Provide focused education for each task the patient or caregiver identifies as having been difficult in terms of moving the patient from the chair to the bathroom.
What questions or concerns do you have regarding moving [patient] from the chair to the bathroom?	Provide specific strategies for overcoming or addressing the challenges the patient or caregiver has encountered when moving the patient from the chair to the bathroom.
	Answer the patient's and caregiver's questions and address their concerns regarding moving the patient from the chair to the bathroom.

MOVING ON/OFF TOILET

Walk me through how you [help patient] get onto and off of the toilet.	Offer concrete praise to the patient and caregiver regarding at least one aspect of the process they've been using to move the patient onto and off of the toilet.
What tasks are the most difficult for you in terms of moving [patient] onto and off of the toilet?	Provide focused education for any tasks that the patient or caregiver has been performing incorrectly (based on their description of the process).
What challenges or problems have you encountered moving [patient] onto and off of the toilet?	Provide focused education for each task the patient or caregiver identifies as having been difficult in terms of moving the patient onto and off of the toilet.
What questions or concerns do you have regarding moving [patient] onto and off of the toilet?	Provide specific strategies for overcoming or addressing the challenges the patient or caregiver has encountered when moving the patient onto and off of the toilet.
	Answer the patient's and caregiver's questions and address their concerns regarding moving the patient onto and off of the toilet.

GETTING IN/OUT OF CAR

Walk me through how you [help patient] get into and out of the car.	Offer concrete praise to the patient and caregiver regarding at least one aspect of the process they've been using to get the patient into and out of the car.
What tasks are the most difficult for you in terms of getting [patient] into and out of the car?	Provide focused education for any tasks that the patient or caregiver has been performing incorrectly (based on their description of the process).

Questions for assessing patient and caregiver knowledge and needs	Addressing knowledge and needs when teaching patient-care skills
What challenges or problems have you encountered getting [patient] into and out of the car? What questions or concerns do you have regarding getting [patient] into and out of the car?	Provide focused education for each task the patient or caregiver identifies as having been difficult in terms of getting the patient into and out of the car. Provide specific strategies for overcoming or addressing the challenges the patient or caregiver has encountered when getting the patient into and out of the car. Answer the patient's and caregiver's questions and address their concerns regarding getting the patient in and out of the car.

MANAGING INCONTINENCE

Walk me through how you [help patient] manage incontinence of urine and stool (accidents, leakage, etc.). What tasks are the most difficult for you in terms of [helping patient] manage incontinence of urine and stool? What challenges or problems have you encountered [helping patient] manage incontinence of urine and stool? What questions or concerns do you have regarding [helping patient] manage incontinence of urine or stool?	Offer concrete praise to the patient and caregiver regarding at least one aspect of the process they've been using to help manage incontinence of urine and stool. Provide focused education for any tasks that the patient or caregiver has been performing incorrectly (based on their description of the process). Provided hands-on instruction to the patient and caregiver regarding the correct use of universal precautions. Provide focused education for each task the patient or caregiver identifies as having been difficult in terms of managing incontinence of urine and stool. Provide specific strategies for overcoming or addressing the challenges the patient or caregiver has encountered in managing incontinence of urine and stool. Answer the patient or caregiver's questions and address their concerns regarding managing incontinence of urine and stool.

NIGHTTIME BATHROOM NEEDS

Walk me through how you [help patient] with nighttime bathroom needs? What tasks are the most difficult for you in terms of [helping patient] with nighttime bathroom needs? What challenges or problems have you encountered [helping patient] with nighttime bathroom needs? What questions or concerns do you have regarding [helping patient] with nighttime bathroom needs?	Offer concrete praise to the patient and caregiver regarding at least one aspect of the process they've been using to help with nighttime bathroom needs. Provide focused education for any tasks that the patient or caregiver has been performing incorrectly (based on their description of the process). Provide focused education for each task the patient or caregiver identifies as having been difficult in terms of helping the patient with nighttime bathroom needs. Provide specific strategies for overcoming or addressing the challenges the patient or caregiver has encountered when helping the patient with nighttime bathroom needs. Answer the patient's and caregiver's questions and address their concerns regarding helping the patient with nighttime bathroom needs.

1. Walk me through how you help [patient] with _____.
   - *Offer concrete praise to the caregiver regarding at least one aspect of the process he or she has been following to help the patient. Provide focused education to correct any tasks the caregiver has been performing incorrectly (based on the caregiver's description of the process).*
2. What tasks are the most difficult for you in terms of helping [patient] with _____?
   - *Provide focused education for each task the caregiver identifies as having been difficult.*
3. What challenges or problems have you encountered helping [patient] with _____?
   - *Provide specific strategies for overcoming or addressing the challenges the caregiver has encountered.*
4. What questions or concerns do you have regarding helping [patient] with _____?
   - *Answer the caregiver's questions and address the caregiver's concerns.*

HOW TO ASSESS KNOWLEDGE AND TEACH ABOUT END-STAGE DISEASE PROGRESSION

When assessing the patient's and caregiver's knowledge regarding a particular aspect of **end-stage disease progression**, keep things simple by asking just one question. For example: "What have you heard about recurrent infections in someone with [patient's] diagnosis and what they mean in terms of the progression of the disease?" The patient's and caregiver's answers will give you a good jumping-off point for focused education. Table 8.2 walks you through the process of assessing patient and caregiver knowledge and addressing knowledge gaps related to end-stage disease progression. Because the particulars of end-stage disease progression will depend on the patient's primary diagnosis, you should omit or add questions, depending on your professional judgment as a physician, APRN, or RN.

TABLE 8.2   ASSESSING AND TEACHING ABOUT
END-STAGE DISEASE PROGRESSION

End-stage disease progression	Questions for assessing patient and caregiver knowledge and needs	Addressing knowledge and needs when teaching about end-stage disease progression
CLINICAL STATUS		
Repeated or intractable infections, such as pneumonia, sepsis, or upper urinary tract [infection]	What have you heard about repeated infections in someone with [patient's] diagnosis and what they mean in terms of the progression of the disease?	Provide focused education to address myths, misinformation, and knowledge gaps about repeated infections and their significance as indicators of end-stage disease progression.
Weight loss not due to reversible causes such as depression or use of diuretics	What have you heard about weight loss in someone with [patient's] diagnosis and what it means in terms of the progression of the disease?	Provide focused education to address myths, misinformation, and knowledge gaps about weight loss and its significance as an indicator of end-stage disease progression.
Dysphagia leading to recurrent aspiration and/or inadequate oral intake documented by decreasing food portion consumption	What have you heard about swallowing problems (dysphagia) in someone with [patient's] diagnosis and what that means in terms of the progression of the disease?	Provide focused education to address myths, misinformation, and knowledge gaps about swallowing problems and their significance as indicators of end-stage disease progression.
SYMPTOMS		
Dyspnea with increasing respiratory rate	What have you heard about shortness of breath or breathlessness (dyspnea) in someone with [patient's] diagnosis and what it means in terms of the progression of the disease?	Provide focused education to address myths, misinformation, and knowledge gaps about shortness of breath or breathlessness and its significance as an indicator of end-stage disease progression.
Intractable coughing	What have you heard about coughing that won't go away in someone with [patient's diagnosis] and what it means in terms of the progression of the disease?	Provide focused education to address myths, misinformation, and knowledge gaps about intractable coughing and its significance as an indicator of end-stage disease progression.
Nausea/vomiting poorly responsive to treatment	What have you heard about nausea/vomiting that won't go away in someone with [patient's] diagnosis and what it means in terms of the progression of the disease?	Provide focused education to address myths, misinformation, and knowledge gaps about nausea/vomiting that won't go away and its significance as an indicator of end-stage disease progression.

continued

End-stage disease progression	Questions for assessing patient and caregiver knowledge and needs	Addressing knowledge and needs when teaching about end-stage disease progression
Intractable diarrhea	What have you heard about diarrhea that won't go away in someone with [patient's] diagnosis and what it means in terms of the progression of the disease?	Provide focused education to address myths, misinformation, and knowledge gaps about intractable diarrhea and its significance as an indicator of end-stage disease progression.
Pain requiring increasing doses of major analgesics more than briefly	What have you heard about pain that requires increasing doses of pain medication in someone with [patient's] diagnosis and what it means in terms of the progression of the disease?	Provide focused education to address myths, misinformation, and knowledge gaps about pain that requires increasing doses of pain medication and its significance as an indicator of end-stage disease progression.
SIGNS		
Decline in systolic blood pressure to below 90, or progressive postural hypotension	What have you heard about low blood pressure or dizziness when standing up in someone with [patient's] diagnosis and what it means in terms of the progression of the disease?	Provide focused education to address myths, misinformation, and knowledge gaps about low blood pressure or dizziness when standing up and its significance as an indicator of end-stage disease progression.
Ascites	What have you heard about abdominal swelling (ascites) in someone with [patient's] diagnosis and what it means in terms of the progression of the disease?	Provide focused education to address myths, misinformation, and knowledge gaps about abdominal swelling and its significance as an indicator of end-stage disease progression.
Venous, arterial, or lymphatic obstruction due to local progression or metastatic disease	What have you heard about obstructions in veins, arteries, or the lymphatic system in someone with [patient's] diagnosis and what they mean in terms of the progression of the disease?	Provide focused education to address myths, misinformation, and knowledge gaps about obstructions in veins, arteries, or the lymphatic system and their significance as indicators of end-stage disease progression.
Edema	What have you heard about swelling (edema) in someone with [patient's] diagnosis and what it means in terms of the progression of the disease?	Provide focused education to address myths, misinformation, and knowledge gaps about swelling (edema) and its significance as an indicator of end-stage disease progression.

End-stage disease progression	Questions for assessing patient and caregiver knowledge and needs	Addressing knowledge and needs when teaching about end-stage disease progression
Pleural/pericardial effusion	What have you heard about pleural/pericardial effusion in someone with [patient's] diagnosis and what it means in terms of the progression of the disease?	Provide focused education to address myths, misinformation, and knowledge gaps about pleural/pericardial effusion and its significance as an indicator of end-stage disease progression.
Weakness	What have you heard about weakness in someone with [patient's] diagnosis and what it means in terms of the progression of the disease?	Provide focused education to address myths, misinformation, or knowledge gaps about weakness and its significance as an indicator of end-stage disease progression.
Change in level of consciousness	What have you heard about changes in the level of consciousness in someone with [patient's] diagnosis and what they mean in terms of the progression of the disease?	Provide focused education to address myths, misinformation, and knowledge gaps about changes in the level of consciousness and their significance as indicators of end-stage disease progression.
OTHER INDICATORS		
Increasing emergency room visits, hospitalizations, or physician's visits related to primary diagnosis	What have you heard about repeated emergency room visits or hospitalizations in someone with [patient's] diagnosis and what they mean in terms of the progression of the disease?	Provide focused education to address myths, misinformation, and knowledge gaps about repeated emergency room visits or hospitalizations and their significance as indicators of end-stage disease progression
Progression to dependence on assistance with additional activities of daily living	What have you heard about increased dependence on help for activities of daily living in someone with [patient's] diagnosis and what it means in terms of the progression of the disease?	Provide focused education to address myths, misinformation, and knowledge gaps about increased dependence on help for activities of daily living and its significance as an indicator of end-stage disease progression.
Progressive stage 3–4 pressure ulcers in spite of optimal care	What have you heard about pressure ulcers in someone with [patient's] diagnosis and what they mean in terms of the progression of the disease?	Provide focused education to address myths, misinformation, and knowledge gaps about pressure ulcers and their significance as indicators of end-stage disease progression.

[a] Text under "End-stage disease progression" is from Centers for Medicaid and Medicare Services 2015a. Reprinted with permission.

HOW TO ASSESS KNOWLEDGE AND TEACH ABOUT PAIN AND SYMPTOM MANAGEMENT

When you teach a patient and caregiver about pain and symptom management, start by reviewing the patient's answers to questions in Dimension 3 of the Five-Dimension Assessment Model. Table 8.3 explains how to assess the patient's and caregiver's prior knowledge of pain and symptom management and then teach them what they need to know.

HOW TO ASSESS KNOWLEDGE AND TEACH ABOUT MEDICATION MANAGEMENT

To manage medications effectively, patients and caregivers need to have a core set of skills: "management skills such as the ability to store, organize, and discard medications, and technical skills such as the ability to recognize symptoms and administer different types of medications" (Lau et al. 2009). Teaching these core skills to patients and caregivers not only facilitates safe and effective **medication management** but also helps you comply with insurance and regulatory requirements. When you document in the patient's medical record the education and training you have provided, you give others a clear picture of the actions taken to ensure that both patient and family are equipped to administer the medications prescribed.

Before you can begin teaching the patient and caregiver how to manage the patient's medications, you need to have a clear understanding of what those medications are and, in the case of a recent or impending care transition, any changes in the medications. This understanding can by attained through the process of **medication reconciliation,** which involves "creating the most accurate list possible of all medications a patient is taking—including drug name, dosage, frequency, and route—and comparing that list against the [clinician's] admission, transfer, and/or discharge orders, with the goal of providing correct medications to the patient at all transition points" (Institute for Healthcare Improvement 2016). For a detailed guide to medication reconciliation, see *Medications*

TABLE 8.3 **ASSESSING AND TEACHING ABOUT PAIN AND SYMPTOM MANAGEMENT**

Questions for assessing patient and caregiver knowledge and needs	Addressing knowledge and needs when teaching about pain and symptom management
ANXIETY	
How can you tell when [patient] is experiencing anxiety? What have you tried in the past to help [patient] with anxiety? What challenges or problems have you encountered in helping [patient] with anxiety? What questions or concerns do you have regarding [patient's] anxiety?	Provide focused education on preventing and addressing anxiety using both nonpharmacologic and pharmacologic approaches, as prescribed by the patient's primary care provider. Provide specific strategies for overcoming or addressing challenges the patient and caregiver have encountered in helping the patient with anxiety. Answer the patient's and caregiver's questions and address their concerns regarding helping the patient with anxiety.
BREATHLESSNESS	
How can you tell when [patient] is experiencing breathlessness? What have you tried in the past to help [patient] with breathlessness? What challenges or problems have you encountered in helping [patient] with breathlessness? What questions or concerns do you have regarding [patient's] breathlessness?	Provide focused education on preventing and addressing breathlessness using both nonpharmacologic and pharmacologic approaches, as prescribed by the patient's primary care provider. Provide specific strategies for overcoming or addressing challenges the patient and caregiver have encountered in helping the patient with breathlessness. Answer the patient's and caregiver's questions and address their concerns regarding helping the patient with breathlessness.
CONFUSION	
How can you tell when [patient] is experiencing confusion? What have you tried in the past to help [patient] with confusion? What challenges or problems have you encountered in helping [patient] with confusion? What questions or concerns do you have regarding [patient's] confusion?	Provide focused education on preventing and addressing confusion using both nonpharmacologic and pharmacologic approaches, as prescribed by the patient's primary care provider. Provide specific strategies for overcoming or addressing challenges the patient and caregiver have encountered in helping the patient with confusion. Answer the patient's and caregiver's questions and address their concerns regarding helping the patient with confusion.
CONSTIPATION	
How can you tell when [patient] is experiencing constipation? What have you tried in the past to help [patient] with constipation?	Provide focused education regarding preventing and addressing constipation using both nonpharmacologic and pharmacologic approaches, as prescribed by the patient's primary care provider.

continued

Questions for assessing patient and caregiver knowledge and needs	Addressing knowledge and needs when teaching about pain and symptom management
What challenges or problems have you encountered in helping [patient] with constipation? What questions or concerns do you have regarding [patient's] constipation?	Provide specific strategies for overcoming or addressing challenges the patient and caregiver have encountered in helping the patient with constipation. Answer the patient's and caregiver's questions and address their concerns regarding helping the patient with constipation.
DEPRESSION	
How can you tell when [patient] is experiencing depression? What have you tried in the past to help [patient] with depression? What challenges or problems have you encountered in helping [patient] with depression? What questions or concerns do you have regarding [patient's] depression?	Provide focused education regarding preventing and addressing depression using both nonpharmacologic and pharmacologic approaches, as prescribed by the patient's primary care provider. Provide specific strategies for overcoming or addressing challenges the patient and caregiver have encountered in helping the patient with depression. Answer the patient's and caregiver's questions and address their concerns regarding helping the patient with depression.
INSOMNIA	
How can you tell when [patient] is experiencing insomnia? What have you tried in the past to help [patient] with insomnia? What challenges or problems have you encountered in helping [patient] with insomnia? What questions or concerns do you have regarding [patient's] insomnia?	Provide focused education on preventing and addressing insomnia using both nonpharmacologic and pharmacologic approaches, as prescribed by the patient's primary care provider. Provide specific strategies for overcoming or addressing challenges the patient and caregiver have encountered in helping the patient with insomnia. Answer the patient's and caregiver's questions and address their concerns regarding helping the patient with insomnia.
NAUSEA/VOMITING	
How can you tell when [patient] is experiencing nausea or vomiting? What have you tried in the past to help [patient] with nausea or vomiting? What challenges or problems have you encountered in helping [patient] with nausea or vomiting? What questions or concerns do you have regarding [patient's] nausea or vomiting?	Provide focused education on preventing and addressing nausea/vomiting using both nonpharmacologic and pharmacologic approaches, as prescribed by the patient's primary care provider. Provide hands-on instruction to the patient and caregiver in the correct universal precautions to follow when there is a risk of exposure to blood or body fluids. Provide specific strategies for overcoming or addressing challenges the patient and caregiver have encountered in helping the patient with nausea/vomiting. Answer the patient's and caregiver's questions and address their concerns regarding helping the patient with nausea/vomiting.

Questions for assessing patient and caregiver knowledge and needs	Addressing knowledge and needs when teaching about pain and symptom management
WEAKNESS/FATIGUE	
How can you tell when [patient] is experiencing weakness or fatigue? What have you tried in the past to help [patient] with weakness or fatigue? What challenges or problems have you encountered in helping [patient] with weakness or fatigue? What questions or concerns do you have regarding [patient's] weakness or fatigue?	Provide focused education on preventing and addressing weakness and fatigue using both nonpharmacologic and pharmacologic approaches, as prescribed by the patient's primary care provider. Provide specific strategies for overcoming or addressing challenges the patient and caregiver have encountered in helping the patient with weakness and fatigue. Answer the patient's and caregiver's questions and address their concerns regarding helping the patient with weakness and fatigue.
WEIGHT LOSS	
How can you tell when [patient] is experiencing weight loss? What have you tried in the past to address [patient's] weight loss? What challenges or problems have you encountered in addressing [patient's] weight loss? What questions or concerns do you have regarding [patient's] weight loss?	Provide focused education on preventing and addressing weight loss using both nonpharmacologic and pharmacologic approaches, as prescribed by the patient's primary care provider. Provide specific strategies for overcoming or addressing challenges the patient and caregiver have encountered in helping the patient with weight loss. Answer the patient's and caregiver's questions and address their concerns regarding helping the patient with weight loss.
PAIN	
How can you tell when [patient] is experiencing pain? What have you tried in the past to help [patient] with pain? What challenges or problems have you encountered in helping [patient] with pain? What questions or concerns do you have regarding [patient's] pain?	Provide focused education on preventing and addressing pain using both nonpharmacologic and pharmacologic approaches, as prescribed by the patient's primary care provider. Provide specific strategies for overcoming or addressing challenges the patient and caregiver have encountered in helping the patient with pain. Answer the patient's and caregiver's questions and address their concerns regarding helping the patient with pain.

at Transitions and Clinical Handoffs (MATCH) Toolkit for Medication Reconciliation (Gleason et al. 2012).

Table 8.4 covers how to assess the patient's and caregiver's knowledge of medication management and address any knowledge gaps. Because the particulars of medication management will depend on the patient's diagnosis, you should omit or add questions as necessary, following your professional judgment as a physician, advanced practice registered nurse, or registered nurse.

HOW TO ASSESS KNOWLEDGE AND TEACH ABOUT DISPOSAL OF SUPPLIES

Table 8.5 walks you through the process of assessing patients' and caregivers' knowledge about how to dispose of medical supplies. It discusses how to address their knowledge gaps and teach them proper procedures related to disposing of supplies such as used syringes and lancets, soiled incontinence pads, and used gauze and bandages.

HOW TO ASSESS KNOWLEDGE AND TEACH ABOUT SIGNS AND SYMPTOMS OF IMMINENT DEATH

Think back to the first time you saw a person die. In the minutes before they took their last breath, did you know what to expect? Or did you have questions you wished you could have asked someone? Were there moments when the person made a noise or a facial expression or movement that frightened or confused you? Your answers to these questions will likely differ depending on whether the first person you saw die was a patient or a close friend or family member.

When patients and families are dealing with a life-limiting illness, fear of the unknown, especially regarding the signs of imminent death, can be distressing. By demystifying the dying process and providing concrete information about what to expect, you can reduce the family's fear and help the patient and family prepare themselves emotionally for the end of life. Table 8.6 is designed to help you assess patient

TABLE 8.4   ASSESSING AND TEACHING ABOUT MEDICATION MANAGEMENT

Skill area	Questions for assessing patient and caregiver knowledge and needs	Addressing knowledge and needs when teaching about medication management
Storing medication	Have you ever used this medication before? If so, where did you keep the medicine? What have you been told about how to store this medication? What questions or concerns do you have about storing this medication?	Provide focused education on how and where to store the medication. Ensure that patient and family understand the precautions they need to take to keep the medication out of reach of children, pets, and others who should not have access to it. Address myths, misinformation, and knowledge gaps about how and where to store the medication. Answer the patient's and caregiver's questions and address their concerns about how and where to store the medication.
Organizing medication	What have you tried in the past to help organize and keep track of [patient's] medications? What challenges or problems have you encountered in organizing and keeping track of [patient's] medications in the past? What questions or concerns do you have regarding organizing and keeping track of [patient's] medications?	Provide focused education on how to organize and keep track of the patient's medications. Consider the patient's and caregiver's literacy level, visual acuity, and cognitive abilities when suggesting tools and strategies. Provide specific strategies for overcoming or addressing challenges the patient and caregiver have encountered in organizing and keeping track of medications. Answer the patient's and caregiver's questions and address their concerns about organizing
Discarding medication	How have you discarded unused medication in the past? What challenges or problems have you encountered in discarding [patient's] medications? What questions or concerns do you have regarding discarding [patient's] medications?	Provide focused education on the proper way to discard medications. Address misinformation and knowledge gaps about safe medication disposal. Ensure that patient and family understand the precautions they need to take to keep discarded medication out of reach of children, pets, and others who should not have access to it.
Administering breakthrough medication	Walk me through/show me the process you use to administer [patient's] breakthrough medication for pain.	Provide focused education for any tasks that the patient or caregiver has been performing incorrectly (based on their description of the process).

continued

Skill area	Questions for assessing patient and caregiver knowledge and needs	Addressing knowledge and needs when teaching about medication management
	What challenges or problems have you encountered in administering [patient's] break-through medication for pain?	Provide specific strategies for overcoming or addressing the challenges the patient or caregiver has encountered in giving breakthrough medication for pain.
	What questions or concerns do you have about administering [patient's] breakthrough medication for pain?	Answer the patient's and caregiver's questions and address their concerns about administering breakthrough medication for pain.
Administering medication patches	Walk me through/show me the process you use to administer [give patient] a medication patch.	Provide focused education for any tasks that the patient or caregiver has been performing incorrectly (based on their description of the process).
	What challenges or problems have you encountered in using [giving patient] a medication patch?	Provide specific strategies for overcoming or addressing challenges the patient or caregiver has encountered with medication patches in the past.
	What questions or concerns do you have regarding using [giving patient] a medication patch?	Answer the patient's and caregiver's questions and address their concerns regarding medication patch use.
Using a syringe	Walk me through/show me the process you use to administer [patient's] medication using a syringe.	Provide focused education for any tasks that the patient or caregiver has been performing incorrectly (based on their description of the process).
	What challenges or problems have you encountered in administering [patient's] medication using a syringe?	Provide hands-on instruction in the correct universal precautions to follow when there is a risk of exposure to blood or body fluids.
	What questions or concerns do you have about administering [patient's] medication using a syringe?	Provide specific strategies for overcoming or addressing challenges the patient or caregiver has encountered in administering medication using a syringe.
		Answer the patient's and caregiver's questions and address their concerns regarding administering medication using a syringe.
Using a dropper	Walk me through/show me the process you use to administer [patient's] medication using a dropper.	Provide focused education for any tasks that the patient or caregiver has been performing incorrectly (based on their description of the process).

Skill area	Questions for assessing patient and caregiver knowledge and needs	Addressing knowledge and needs when teaching about medication management
	What challenges or problems have you encountered in administering [patient's] medication using a dropper? What questions or concerns do you have regarding administering [patient's] medication using a dropper?	Provide specific strategies for overcoming or addressing challenges the patient or caregiver has encountered in administering medication using a dropper. Answer the patient's and caregiver's questions and address their concerns regarding giving medication using a dropper.
Administering pills and capsules	Walk me through/show me the process you use when you administer [patient's] pills and capsules. What challenges or problems have you encountered in administering [patient's] pills and capsules? What questions or concerns do you have regarding administering [patient's] pills and capsules?	Provide focused education for any tasks that the patient or caregiver has been performing incorrectly (based on their description of the process). Provide specific strategies for overcoming or addressing challenges the patient or caregiver has encountered in administering pills and capsules. Answer the patient's and caregiver's questions and address their concerns regarding administering pills and capsules.

and caregiver knowledge of the signs and symptoms of imminent death and then offer information to address their knowledge gaps.

Depending on the patient's primary diagnosis, you may want to provide additional information about what to expect when the patient is dying. For example, if a patient is likely to experience exsanguination or hemoptysis, explain to the patient and family what to expect and consider giving the family several red towels. (Using red towels for cleaning up during and after bleeding can help caregivers avoid or minimize the distressing sight of their loved one's blood.) Be alert to the possibility of exsanguination in patients with ear, nose, or throat tumors; neck metastases; leukemia; bladder tumors; disseminated intravascular coagulation (DIC); or gastrointestinal tumors. While massive hemoptysis is relatively rare, it is a possibility with some types of cancer (Akinola, Baru, and Marks 2015).

TABLE 8.5 ASSESSING AND TEACHING ABOUT DISPOSAL OF SUPPLIES

Skill area	Questions for assessing patient and caregiver knowledge and needs	Addressing knowledge and needs when teaching about disposal of supplies
Disposing of used incontinence pads, diapers, and other supplies soiled with urine and/or stool	How have you disposed of used supplies soiled with urine and/or stool? What challenges or problems have you encountered in disposing of used supplies soiled with urine and/or stool? What questions or concerns do you have about disposing of used supplies soiled with urine and/or stool?	Provide focused education and address knowledge gaps regarding the proper disposal of used supplies soiled with urine and/or stool. Ensure that patient and family understand the precautions they need to take in handling and disposing of used supplies soiled with urine and/or stool. Provide patient and family with the supplies needed for proper disposal.
Disposing of gauze, bandages, and other supplies soiled with blood or body fluids	How have you disposed of supplies soiled with blood or body fluids? What challenges or problems have you had encountered in disposing of supplies soiled with blood or body fluids? What questions or concerns do you have regarding the disposal supplies soiled with blood or body fluids?	Provide focused education and address knowledge gaps regarding the proper disposal of gauze, bandages, and other supplies soiled with blood or body fluids. Ensure that patient and family understand the precautions they need to take in handling and disposing of supplies soiled with blood or body fluids. Provide patient and family with the supplies needed for proper disposal.
Disposing of used syringes, lancets, and other sharps	How have you disposed of used syringes, lancets, and other sharps? What challenges or problems have you encountered in disposing of used syringes, lancets, and other sharps? What questions or concerns do you have about disposing of used syringes, lancets, and other sharps?	Provide focused education and address knowledge gaps regarding the proper disposal of used syringes, lancets, and other sharps. Ensure that patient and family understand the precautions they need to take in handling and disposing of used syringes, lancets, and other sharps. Provide patient and family with the supplies needed for proper disposal.

System	Questions for assessing patient and caregiver knowledge and needs	Addressing knowledge and needs when teaching about signs and symptoms of imminent death
Neurological	What have you heard about how a person's alertness, awareness, or thinking might change as death becomes imminent? What questions, concerns, or worries do you have regarding changes in [patient's] alertness, awareness, or thinking as death becomes imminent?	Provide focused education to address myths, misinformation, or knowledge gaps about neurological changes and their significance as indicators of imminent death. Answer the patient's and caregiver's questions and address their concerns about neurological changes.
Integumentary (skin)	What have you heard about how a person's skin might change as death becomes imminent? What questions, concerns, or worries do you have regarding changes in [patient's] skin as death becomes imminent?	Provide focused education to address myths, misinformation, or knowledge gaps about skin changes and their significance as indicators of imminent death. Answer the patient's and caregiver's questions and address their concerns regarding skin changes.
Respiratory	What have you heard about how a person's breathing might change as death becomes imminent? What questions, concerns, or worries do you have regarding changes in [patient's] breathing as death becomes imminent?	Provide focused education to address myths, misinformation, or knowledge gaps about respiratory changes and their significance as indicators of imminent death. Answer the patient's and caregiver's questions and address their concerns regarding respiratory changes.
Cardiovascular and circulatory	What have you heard about how a person's heart function and circulation might change as death becomes imminent? What questions, concerns, or worries do you have regarding changes in [patient's] heart function or circulation as death becomes imminent?	Provide focused education to address myths, misinformation, or knowledge gaps about cardiac and circulatory changes and their significance as indicators of imminent death. Answer the patient's and caregiver's questions and address their concerns regarding cardiac and circulatory changes.

continued

System	Questions for assessing patient and caregiver knowledge and needs	Addressing knowledge and needs when teaching about signs and symptoms of imminent death
Excretory	What have you heard about how a person's excretion of urine and/or feces might change as death becomes imminent? What questions, concerns, or worries do you have regarding changes in [patient's] excretion of urine and/or feces as death becomes imminent?	Provide focused education to address myths, misinformation, or knowledge gaps about excretory changes and their significance as indicators of imminent death. Answer the patient's and caregiver's questions and address their concerns regarding excretory changes.
Digestive	What have you heard about how a person's desire and ability to eat and drink might change as death becomes imminent? What questions, concerns, or worries do you have regarding changes in [patient's] eating and drinking as death becomes imminent?	Provide focused education to address myths, misinformation, or knowledge gaps about changes in food and fluid intake and their significance as indicators of imminent death. Answer the patient's and caregiver's questions and address their concerns regarding changes in food and fluid intake.

KEY POINTS TO REMEMBER

- Patient and family education is an essential part of the delivery of quality care (Institute of Medicine 2013).
- Patient-care skills are the skills needed by a patient and/or caregiver to support the patient in meeting bathing, dressing, feeding, transferring, toileting, and transportation needs.
- When assessing the caregiver's knowledge of and need for a particular patient-care skill, ask four key questions:
  1. Walk me through how you help [patient] with _____.
  2. What tasks are the most difficult for you in terms of helping [patient] with _____?
  3. What challenges or problems have you encountered in helping [patient] with _____?
  4. What questions or concerns do you have regarding helping [patient] with _____?

- Medication management requires skills on the part of a patient and/or caregiver to store, organize, discard, and administer the patient's medications safely and effectively. Teaching patients and families how to manage medication is usually the role of the physician, APRN, or RN.
- Pain and symptom management requires skills on the part of a patient and/or caregiver to assess and address symptoms including, but not limited to, anxiety, breathlessness, confusion, constipation, depression, insomnia, nausea/vomiting, pain, weakness/fatigue, and weight loss. Teaching patients and families how to manage pain and other symptoms is usually the role of the physician, APRN, or RN, but other members of the team may provide education regarding nonpharmacologic interventions, such as relaxation techniques, mindfulness, meditation, and so on.
- Disposing of supplies—such as used syringes and lancets, soiled incontinence pads, and used gauze and bandages—safely and effectively requires skills on the part of the patient and/or caregiver. Teaching patients and families how to dispose of supplies is generally the role of the physician, APRN, or RN.
- When patients and families are dealing with a life-limiting illness, fear of the unknown regarding end-stage disease progress and signs of imminent death can be distressing. Patient and family education can reduce fear and help the patient and family prepare themselves emotionally for the end of life.

DISCUSSION QUESTIONS

1. How would you assess knowledge of and teach *patient-care skills* to a patient and caregiver? Describe the questions you would ask and explain how your process would vary depending on whether you met with the patient and caregiver together or separately.
2. How would you assess knowledge and teach about *end-*

stage disease progression? Describe the questions you would ask a patient and caregiver and explain how your process would vary depending on whether you met with the patient and caregiver together or separately.

3. How would you assess knowledge and teach about *pain and symptom management?* Describe the questions you would ask and explain how your process would vary depending on whether you met with the patient and caregiver together or separately.

4. How would you assess knowledge and teach about *medication management?* Describe the questions you would ask a patient and their caregiver and explain how your process would vary depending on whether you met with the patient and caregiver together or separately.

5. How would you assess knowledge and teach about the *disposal of supplies?* Describe the questions you would ask a patient and caregiver and explain how your process would vary depending on whether you met with the patient and caregiver together or separately.

6. How would you assess knowledge and teach about the *signs and symptoms of imminent death?* Describe the questions you would ask a patient and caregiver and explain how your process would vary depending on whether you met with the patient and caregiver together or separately.

CHAPTER ACTIVITY

Using the information in this chapter, assess a patient's knowledge and teach the patient about pain and symptom management. (You may work with either a real patient or a simulated patient via role playing.) Immediately afterward, write down your **reflections** on the process. If you used this process in your work with all patients, do you think it would improve the quality of care you deliver? Why or why not?

CHAPTER 9

PSYCHOSOCIAL AND SPIRITUAL ISSUES

CHAPTER OBJECTIVES

1. Describe psychosocial assessment, supportive techniques, and your role as an interdisciplinary/interprofessional team member in using them.
2. Describe emotional distress and strategies for assessing it.
3. List the developmental tasks involved in life completion and life closure.
4. Define despair, hope, and meaning in the context of chronic and life-limiting illness.
5. Describe a spiritual/existential assessment and your role as an interdisciplinary/interprofessional team member in conducting one.
6. Describe common experiences of distress around spiritual/existential issues for patients and families facing chronic and life-limiting conditions.

Key Terms: despair, emotional distress, hope, life completion and life closure, meaning, psychosocial assessment, spiritual/existential assessment, spiritual/existential distress, supportive techniques

Acquaviva, Kimberly
LGBTQ-Inclusive Hospice and Palliative Care
dx.doi.org/10.17312/harringtonparkpress/2017.03lgbtqihpc.009
© 2017 by Kimberly Acquaviva

Assessing and addressing psychosocial and spiritual issues is as important to the delivery of quality care as assessing and addressing pain and other physical symptoms. This chapter explains the developmental tasks of life completion and life closure as well as the roles that despair, hope, and meaning play in the context of advanced illness. The chapter describes LGBTQ-inclusive assessment skills and supportive techniques for addressing psychosocial and spiritual issues, and explains how a spiritual/existential history and a spiritual/existential assessment differ. Finally, the chapter examines the ways in which the members of the interdisciplinary/interprofessional team collaborate to support the patient and family in achieving their goals for care in the psychosocial and spiritual/existential domains.

PSYCHOSOCIAL ASSESSMENT AND SUPPORTIVE TECHNIQUES

Clinical Practice Guidelines for Quality Palliative Care provides guidance regarding the essential elements of psychosocial assessment and support in two areas: the psychological and psychiatric domain (Domain 3 in the guidelines), and the social domain (Domain 4) (National Consensus Project for Quality Palliative Care 2013). The Five-Dimension Assessment Model described in Chapter 4 translates many of the core elements from *Clinical Practice Guidelines for Quality Palliative Care* into a clear and comprehensive list of questions to ask of patients and families when taking an initial history. Psychosocial assessment questions are interwoven throughout the five dimensions to reinforce the practice among interdisciplinary/interprofessional team members of recognizing the interrelated nature of physical and psychosocial issues. Although **psychosocial assessment** is a term used to describe "an evaluation of a person's mental health, social status, and functional capacity within the community, generally conducted by . . . social workers" (*Mosby's Medical Dictionary* 2009), physicians, advanced practice registered nurses, registered nurses, and chaplains may also assess and document the patient's and family's psychosocial issues, stressors, strengths, and goals. Similarly, while supportive psychotherapy is considered to be the domain of licensed mental health practitioners, supportive techniques can be used appropriately and effectively by all members of the patient's interdisciplinary/interprofessional team. As is the case with all care provided by members of the team, any psychosocial assessments and interventions you use should be guided by the scope of practice for your discipline.

Supportive techniques are valuable in developing a positive therapeutic relationship with patients and families. To infuse supportive techniques into your work, maintain a focus on each patient and family and see them as the owners and drivers of their plan of care. This will reinforce the collaborative nature of your relationship with the patient and family and convey your respect for and acceptance of their goals and preferences.

DOCUMENTING PSYCHOSOCIAL ASSESSMENTS

When patients are receiving palliative care or hospice care they interact with and are assessed by multiple members of the interdisciplinary/interprofessional team, each of whom documents their assessment using the lens and language of their discipline. Within hospice, this may lead to seemingly contradictory documentation that can raise questions in the minds of the Centers for Medicare and Medicaid Services (CMS) employees and contractors who conduct medical reviews of claims submitted for payment (Hilliard 2012). When documenting your psychosocial assessment of patients in hospice care, consider including a notation of your "observations related to the patient's hospice eligibility within the scope of [your] practice" (ibid.). Hilliard suggests following what he calls the **DAROP format** for psychosocial documentation, referring to the format's components: data, action, results, observations, and plan (see DAROP "Format for Psychosocial Documentation").

D—Data: Write what you observed at the beginning of the session and relate it to the hospice diagnosis. Write your assessment of need in this session and the care plan you are addressing. Sentences in this section should start with "patient" or "family," as you are documenting what you saw at the beginning of the session. For example, "Patient was received sitting up in the living room watching television with his wife. He appeared melancholic as evidenced by his flat affect and downcast eyes. He denied pain and stated, "I'm just kind of tired today." Care plans being addressed: altered mood (depression) and anticipatory grief.

A—Action: Write what you did in the session to address the needs you assessed. Sentences in this section should start with your position (e.g., chaplain, social worker, music therapist), as you are documenting your interventions for the patient and/or family. For example, "Social worker assessed patient's mood as depressed and provided supportive counseling, empathetic listening, and validation. Social worker introduced the concept of a legacy project and offered to work with patient and family on documenting the patient's life story. Encouraged life review and reminiscence. Contacted RN case manager, Betty Smith, and reported observations of patient's depression."

R—Results: Write observable outcomes of your actions or interventions. Sentences in this section should start with "patient" or "family," as you are documenting what you observed as the result of your interventions. For example, "While the patient was relatively guarded when asked about his depression and current situation, his affect significantly brightened during life review. His wife shared stories of their courtship 30 years ago, and he joined in the discussion with additional stories. While reminiscing, they held hands and laughed. Overall, the patient continues to struggle with his depressed mood, and when the wife walked the social worker outside at the end of the visit, she shared her concerns for her husband. There were no signs of suicidal ideation. She agreed to a legacy project with him as a coping skill to lift his mood."

O—Observations: Write all observations of physical decline related to the diagnosis. You are answering the question: "Within your scope of practice, what do you see that makes this patient hospice-eligible today?" Sentences in this section should start with "patient," as you are describing your objective and subjective observations of his hospice eligibility. For example, "Patient was utilizing oxygen throughout the visit today, whereas on previous visits he would take it on and off. His feet were swollen and he had them raised on a footstool. He said he gets dizzy when he stands, so he rises slowly. Due to his increased weakness, he said he avoids any activities other than moving from his bed to the living room."

P—Plan: Document your plan for further addressing the patient's needs. For example, "Social worker will visit patient next week to further facilitate a legacy project and will continue to assess his and his wife's needs."

From Hilliard 2012. Reprinted with permission of Russell Hilliard, © 2012 Russell Hilliard. Permission also obtained from the National Hospice and Palliative Care Organization.

The term **emotional distress** denotes "an emotional . . . state of pain, sorrow, misery, suffering, or discomfort" (*Mosby's Medical Dictionary* 2009). Emotional distress is sometimes referred to as **psychological distress:** "a range of symptoms and experiences of a person's internal life that are commonly held to be troubling, confusing, or out of the ordinary" (American Psychiatric Association 2016).

When a patient or family member appears to be experiencing emotional distress, first assess for clinically significant depression and **suicidal ideation**, document the results of your assessment, and take the appropriate actions based on your discipline's scope of practice. Clinically significant depression differs from situational depression and may benefit from pharmacologic intervention. Patients and families receiving palliative care and hospice care may be experiencing significant stressors and thus awareness and assessment are prudent.

Although physicians, APRNs, RNs, chaplains, social workers, and counselors may each assess emotional distress within their respective scope of practice, it is good practice to coordinate with the other members of the interdisciplinary/ interprofessional team so that everyone is on the same page. Patients and family members receiving palliative care and hospice services are already dealing with a flood of information — and feelings — that come with a diagnosis of a serious or life-limiting illness. Having three members of the team each conduct a **comprehensive assessment** of emotional distress on the same day could be overwhelming. Joint assessment visits are one strategy to address this. For example, a chaplain and social worker or counselor might meet with a patient or family member together to assess and address emotional distress. When joint visits are conducted skillfully, patients and families feel as though they are part of a conversation rather than the objects of an assessment.

When assessing emotional distress in a patient or family member, be sensitive to the fact that the perceived source of emotional distress may be a long-standing issue—one that may seem to have nothing to do with the seriousness of the patient's life-limiting illness. Lesbian, gay, bisexual, transgender, gender-nonconforming, queer, and/or questioning individuals (or *any* individual, really) may indicate that relationships with their family of origin are the most distressing aspects of their life. Just because an issue has a long history does not mean it cannot (or should not) be addressed by the palliative care or hospice professional. Ask follow-up questions to discern how you might be able to support the patient or family member with their distress over challenging family relationships.

In providing psychosocial support to patients and families, however, it is important to focus on providing support rather than "therapy" surrounding LGBTQ issues. PFLAG (the organization previously known as Parents, Families, and Friends of Lesbians and Gays) is an excellent resource for patients and families seeking information and support. Its website, www.pflag.org, contains a directory of local chapters as well as a number of helpful resources.

Conversely, do not assume that all lesbian, gay, bisexual, transgender, gender-nonconforming, queer, and/or questioning individuals will be experiencing emotional distress in their relationships with their families of origin. Many LGBTQ individuals have positive, supportive family relationships.

DESPAIR, HOPE, AND MEANING IN THE CONTEXT OF ADVANCED ILLNESS

When you ask patients how they cope with distress, you will probably hear the word *hope* quite a bit. Despair, hope, and meaning all play important roles in patients' and families' experiences of growth in the context of advanced illness. **Hope** is "the belief that what is desired is also possible and that events will turn out for the best . . . [and] the feeling that what one believes will occur" (Gladding 2011). Palliative care patients and families may hope for a cure, for remission, for symptom relief, and/or for continued independence. Hospice patients and families may have similar hopes, although it is normal to see a shift from hope for a cure to hope for the best possible quality of life. Patients and families (families of origin and families of choice) may hope for an affirmation of their relationship with and the presence of God, the Creator, a spirit, or whatever they call the source to which they look for support and guidance. It is up to each patient and family to define what hope means for them. Your role is to offer information, choices, and support, not the permission to hope for a given outcome.

The converse of hope is **despair**, "an inability . . . to find meaning in one's life. . . . A complete loss of hope" (Gladding 2011). Despair is a state of existential angst that arises from the void where hope and meaning used to be. When patients and families experience despair, it's very painful. When a person finds **meaning** in their life, they feel as though their life has "significance and purposefulness" (ibid.). Part of your role is to help patients and families find hope, find meaning, and, ultimately, complete the developmental tasks associated with life completion and life closure.

LIFE COMPLETION AND LIFE CLOSURE: DEVELOPMENTAL TASKS

Individuals facing serious or life-limiting conditions continue to have opportunities for personal growth and fulfillment. Whether you are a physician, social worker, counselor, chaplain, advanced practice registered nurse, or registered nurse, there are things you can do to support patients and families in completing the developmental tasks associated with **life completion and life closure.** Byock's chart "Developmental Landmarks and Taskwork for the End of Life" (1994), reprinted in table 9.1, is a seminal resource that provides a clearly articulated model for the developmental tasks associated with life completion and life closure.

TABLE 9.1   BYOCK'S DEVELOPMENTAL LANDMARKS
AND TASKWORK FOR THE END OF LIFE

Landmarks	Taskwork
Sense of completion with worldly affairs	• Transfer of fiscal, legal, and formal social responsibilities
Sense of completion in relationships with community	• Closure of multiple social relationships (employment, commerce, organizational, congregational); components include: expressions of regret, expressions of forgiveness, acceptance of gratitude and appreciation • Leave taking; the saying of good-bye
Sense of meaning about one's individual life	• Life review • The telling of "one's stories" • Transmission of knowledge and wisdom
Experienced love of self	• Self-acknowledgment • Self-forgiveness
Experienced love of others	• Acceptance of worthiness
Sense of completion in relationships with family and friends	• Reconciliation, fullness of communication, and closure in each of one's important relationships; components include: expressions of regret, expressions of forgiveness and acceptance, expressions of gratitude and appreciation, acceptance of gratitude and appreciation, expressions of affection • Leave-taking; the saying of good-bye
Acceptance of the finality of life—of one's existence as an individual	• Acknowledgment of the totality of personal loss represented by one's dying, and experience of personal pain of existential loss • Expression of the depth of personal tragedy that dying represents • *Decathexis* (emotional withdrawal) from worldly affairs and *cathexis* (emotional connection) with an enduring construct • Acceptance of dependency
Sense of a new self (personhood) beyond personal loss	• Developing self-awareness in the present
Sense of meaning about life in general	• Achieving a sense of awe • Recognition of a transcendent realm • Developing/achieving a sense of comfort with chaos
Surrender to the transcendent, to the unknown— "letting go"	• In pursuit of this landmark, the doer and "taskwork" are one. Here, little remains of the ego except the volition to surrender.

Source: Byock 1994. Reprinted with permission from Ira Byock, MD, © 1994.

So often I hear people say, "Hospice is not about giving up hope," and my response is, "Says who?!" I get that the notion of hope changes, yet I also think that letting go of hope for continued life is something we should be offering to address with patients and families, and that it is likely we do not do this enough. Just because we are not doing psychotherapy based on a clinical diagnosis does not mean we are not using many of the same interventions we would use in psychotherapy or "counseling" sessions. We can be using things like motivational interviewing to create person-centered plans of care; mindfulness techniques to address pain/symptom management, stress, agitation; the dual process model for grief and loss; and much of cognitive behavioral therapy (CBT) can be used by us to help address suffering at all levels. Social workers, counselors, and chaplains can use mindfulness, guided imagery, "combat breathing," and many of the CBT interventions. One of my mantras is, "How do we get beyond active listening and emotional support?" And as Kübler-Ross said, "People are dying here. There is no time for funny business!"

—GARY GARDIA, M.ED, MSW, LCSW

Because Byock's developmental tasks are presented as a list, it can be tempting to imagine them as easily defined tasks on a linear checklist of sorts. However, most of the developmental tasks have no discrete beginning or endpoint. Patients may move in and out of accepting their own worthiness or feeling comfortable with chaos. There is no right or wrong way to progress through these developmental tasks—every patient is unique in how, when, and even if they tackle them. Remember, your role is to be a supportive guide, not a taskmaster.

Using these developmental tasks as an organizing framework, Byock and Merriman developed the Missoula-VITAS Quality of Life Index (MVQOLI), a validated, widely used instrument designed to assess quality of life along the following dimensions:

> **Symptoms (S):** Experience of physical discomfort associated with progressive illness and the resulting level of physical distress; **Functional (F):** Perceived ability to perform accustomed functions and activities of daily living experienced in relation to the person's expectations, and the associated emotional response; **Interpersonal (IP):** Degree of investment in personal relationships and the perceived quality of one's relations/interactions with family and friends; **Well-being (WB):** Self-assessment of a person's internal condition. A subjective sense of wellness or disease, contentment or lack of contentment; **Transcendent (T):** Experienced degree of connection with an enduring construct; degree of experienced meaning and purpose of one's life. (Byock and Merriman 1998)

Although the MVQOLI was originally developed for use with patients facing a terminal, life-limiting illness, "the MVQOLI has been used with palliative care and hospice patients in a variety of settings including hospice, hospital, home health, long-term care (including assisted living), outpatient palliative care, and pre-hospice programs . . . [and] is appropriate for any patient population facing advanced, chronic, progressive illness" (Byock and Merriman n.d.). Consider using the MVQOLI to gain a better understanding of patients' quality of life from a holistic perspective.

SPIRITUAL/EXISTENTIAL ASSESSMENT: WHOSE JOB IS IT?

In palliative care and hospice care, chaplains are the members of the interdisciplinary/interprofessional team with the most training and experience in providing a **spiritual/existential assessment,** "an informed judgment concerning treatment options based on the spiritual [or existential] history" (LaRocca-Pitts 2007). However, other members of the team may conduct spiritual histories or support the patient and family in achieving their goals of care related to spirituality or existential concerns.

All too often, team members ask patients and families only a single screening question in the spiritual arena: "Would you like to see a chaplain?" Instead of asking such a narrow question, consider saying something like this to patients: "Many people I work with say they worry about what will happen to them after they die. Is that something that you've been thinking about?" If the patient's answer is yes, you can respond by saying, "There's someone on our team who's really good with those conversations. Can I have that person call you?" Another way you could open the conversation might include asking, for example, "In times when you experience challenges such as serious illness, what are some ways that you cope and find strength?"

There's a difference between a **spiritual/existential history** and a **spiritual/existential assessment**, although the two terms are often used interchangeably or indistinctly. The text *Clinical Practice Guidelines for Quality Palliative Care*, for example, does not articulate a distinction between spiritual assessment and spiritual history, nor does it distinguish between which members of the team should be able to take such a history and which should be able to design and implement treatment and interventions to address issues identified during the history. A reference is made to people operating only within their scope of practice, but ideally this should be made more explicit: "A spiritual assessment process, including a spiritual screening, history questions, and a full spiritual assessment as indicated, is performed. This assessment identifies religious or spiritual/existential background, preferences, and related beliefs, rituals, and practices of the patient and family; as well as symptoms, such as spiritual distress and/or pain, guilt, resentment, despair, and hopelessness" (National Consensus Project for Quality Palliative Care 2013).

A clearer description of the terms *spiritual history* and *spiritual assessment* can be found in "Improving the Quality of Spiritual Care as a Dimension of Palliative Care: The Report of the Consensus Conference":

> Spiritual history-taking is the process of interviewing a patient in order to come to a better understanding of their spiritual needs and resources. A spiritual history can be integrated into existing formats such as the social history section of the clinical database. . . . The information from the history permits the clinician to understand how spiritual concerns could either complement or complicate the patient's overall care. It also allows the clinician to incorporate spiritual care into the patient's overall care plan. . . . [T]hose doing a spiritual history should have some education in and comfort with issues that may emerge and knowledge of how to engage patients comfortably in this discussion. (Puchalski et al. 2009)

In contrast to a spiritual history, which may be completed by a physician, registered nurse, advanced practice registered nurse, social worker, or chaplain, among others, a spiritual assessment (also called a spiritual/existential assessment) refers to

> a more extensive process of active listening to a patient's story conducted by a board-certified chaplain that summarizes the needs and resources that emerge in that process. The chaplain's summary should include a spiritual care plan with expected outcomes that is then communicated to the rest of the treatment team. Unlike history-taking, the major models for spiritual assessment are not built on a set of questions that can be used in an interview. Rather, the models are interpretive frameworks that are based on listening to the patient's story as it unfolds. Because of the complex nature of these

assessments and the special clinical training necessary to engage in them, this assessment should be done only by a board-certified chaplain or an equivalently prepared spiritual care provider. (Puchalski et al. 2009)

In summary, any member of the team may conduct a spiritual history, but only a board-certified chaplain or spiritual care provider with equivalent training should complete a spiritual assessment.

Figure 9.1, which comes from Puchalski et al. (2009), "Improving the Quality of Spiritual Care as a Dimension of Palliative Care," illustrates how the spiritual history, spiritual assessment, and spiritual interventions and treatment fit together in an inpatient setting. The diagram outlines an approach that would be appropriate in both palliative care and hospice care, regardless of setting.

Note: As you conduct a spiritual history of a patient, remember the mitigation plan discussed in Chapter 1. It is important that you prevent your unconscious biases from having a negative impact on the care you provide to that patient.

THE IMPORTANCE OF INCLUSIVE LANGUAGE

When you ask a patient or patient's family about their spiritual/existential needs, you are asking them to enter into a very personal dialogue with you about a part of their life that may be very important to them. As is the case with every aspect of an assessment, the words you use in opening that conversation can either build a bridge or burn one. Table 9.2 offers a few examples of how the words you use may not convey the message you intend.

The language you use with patients and families should be inclusive enough that they should not be able to guess your own spiritual or religious beliefs. Ask questions in a way that conveys that you are open to all possible answers. The spiritual history questions in Dimension 1-A of the Five-

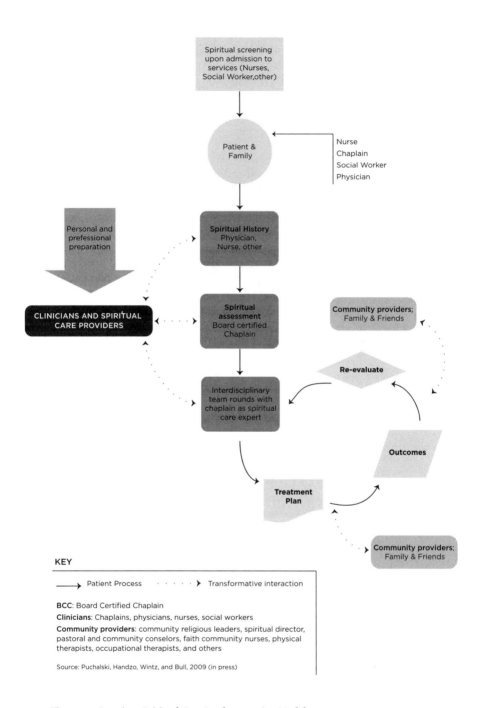

Figure 9.1 Inpatient Spiritual Care Implementation Model
Source: Puchalski et al. 2009. Reprinted with permission of Mary Ann Liebert, Inc., © 2009 Mary Ann Liebert, Inc. The publisher for this copyrighted material is Mary Ann Liebert, Inc.

TABLE 9.2 **INTENT VERSUS IMPACT**

What You Say	What You Imply
"Are you part of a church?"	I can't imagine you'd be anything other than Christian.
"Do you believe in God?"	I have a traditional, narrowly defined concept of spirituality. If you have a more expansive concept of a higher power, I'm probably not going to be receptive to talking with you about it.
"Would you like me to call a priest?"	You're dying—like, soon. And obviously you're Catholic, right?
"I'm guessing from your last name that you're Jewish?"	I am super awkward when it comes to asking questions about spirituality, but I'm trying.

Dimension Assessment Model are examples of open-ended, inclusive questions (see the box "FICA Spiritual History Tool" in Chapter 4).

Inclusive language and open-ended questions are essential to conducting an effective spiritual/existential history (Knight n.d). If you struggle to think outside the box of your own spiritual or religious beliefs, strive to learn more about other spiritual and religious beliefs and traditions. The more you learn about other ways of making sense of the world spiritually and existentially, the more comfortable you will be eliciting spiritual/existential histories from patients and families.

COMMON EXPERIENCES OF SPIRITUAL/ EXISTENTIAL DISTRESS

Feelings of **spiritual/existential distress** may consist of "discomfort related to religious, intellectual, or cultural concerns" or "a disruption in the life principle that pervades a person's entire being and that integrates and transcends his or her biological and psychosocial nature" (*Miller-Keane Encyclopedia and Dictionary of Medicine* 2003). When patients or family

There they were. The old church lady and the young man with the purse. Sitting next to each other at the Sunday afternoon worship service I coordinated at the hospice home. "This will never work," I thought. She, a conservative Christian of many years; he, a lapsed Catholic of many fewer years. Her gray hair was adorned by a little hat with a veil, all black and gray, like her attire. His head was bare, but his outfit was brightly colored. The only thing similar about them was that they both smelled of floral perfume—hers understated, his discernible across the room. Quietly I prayed for a miracle: that they would get along, just this once, as they sat together. I needn't have worried. Every week they came to service, and sat next to each other. In fact, they became the best of friends. Sure, the differences were many. But what they had in common was that they were both dying, or—better said—living until they died. They both sought God in their own way and found him to be bigger, together, than I had imagined possible. As they shared that experience, they formed a bond of friendship that taught me that important lesson.

—STEVE SHICK, MDIV, MA REL, BCC

members experience spiritual/existential distress, they may voice "concern[s] with the meaning of life and death, question the meaning of suffering or of [their] own existence, verbalize inner conflict about beliefs, express **anger** toward God or other Supreme Being (however defined), or actively seek spiritual assistance" (ibid.).

Any patient or family member may experience spiritual/existential distress, including patients who have had very negative experiences with religion in the past. A transgender patient raised in an Orthodox Jewish family, for example, may have spent her life hearing messages that the male sex she was assigned at birth will be her "halachic gender"—her gender according to Jewish law—for life (Kaleem 2016). When this patient is facing a chronic or life-limiting illness, she may struggle with those messages replaying on a loop in her head and feel conflicted about her decision to stop wearing tefillin when she transitioned to her true gender. She may struggle to reconcile her own beliefs with the beliefs she was taught as a child. This is not only the case with LGBTQ individuals—heterosexual and cisgender individuals may struggle with these issues as well.

Spiritual distress may manifest itself in a variety of a ways, many of which may seem to overlap with indicators of psychosocial or emotional distress. In "Improving the Quality of Spiritual Care as a Dimension of Palliative Care: The Report of the Consensus Conference," Puchalski and colleagues (2009) illustrate the connections between specific spiritual "diagnoses" and the way they are manifested through a patient's or family member's history and statements (see table 9.3).

SUPPORTING THOSE IN SPIRITUAL/EXISTENTIAL DISTRESS

Physician Daniel Sulmasy argues that there are three "pressing categories of spiritual questions that serious illness raises—questions of meaning, value, and relationship" (Sulmasy 2006). To help patients and families make meaning of their experience, Sulmasy suggests that clinicians ask them questions in each of the three areas. Sulmasy's final question—"If you're a religious person, how are things between you and God?"—represents a somewhat narrow conceptualization of what it means to be a "religious person." People may consider themselves to be religious and yet not believe in the existence of a solitary deity named "God." Rather than posing the question Sulmasy suggests, try asking something like, "If you believe in a higher power—a guiding force, deity, God,

TABLE 9.3 SPIRITUAL CONCERNS

Diagnosis (primary)	Key feature from history	Example statements
Existential Concerns	Lack of meaning Questions the meaning about one's own existence Concern about afterlife Questions the meaning of suffering Seeks spiritual assistance	"My life is meaningless." "I feel useless."
Abandonment by God or others	Lack of love, loneliness Not being remembered No sense of relatedness	"God has abandoned me." "No one comes by anymore."
Anger at God or others	Displaces anger toward religious representatives Inability to forgive	"Why would God take my child...it's not fair."
Concerns about relationship with deity	Desires closeness to God, deepening relationship	"I want to have a deeper relationship with God."
Conflicted or challenged belief systems	Verbalizes inner conflicts or questions about beliefs or faith Conflicts between religious beliefs and recommended treatments Questions moral or ethical implications of therapeutic regimen Expresses concern with life/death or belief system	"I am not sure if God is with me anymore."
Despair / Hopelessness	Hopelessness about future health, life Despair as absolute hopelessness No hope for value in life	"Life is being cut short." "There is nothing left for me to live for."
Grief / loss	The feeling and process associated with the loss of a person, health, relationship	"I miss my loved one so much." "I wish I could run again."
Guilt / Shame	Feeling that one has done something wrong or evil Feeling that one is bad or evil	"I do not deserve to die pain-free."
Reconciliation	Need for forgiveness or reconciliation from self or others	"I need to be forgiven for what I did." "I would like my wife to forgive me."
Isolation	Separated from religious community or others	"Since moving to the assisted living I am not able to go to my church anymore."
Religious-specific	Ritual needs Unable to perform usual religious practices	"I just can't pray anymore."
Religious / spiritual struggle	Loss of faith or meaning Religious or spiritual beliefs or community not helping with coping	"What if all that I believe is not true."

The story I will share with you is not my proudest moment, but it's one that taught me a great deal. We had a home hospice patient who had identified herself to the RN case manager on the home team as a transgender person named Susan. When I called to introduce spiritual care and schedule a visit, I overlooked that note and addressed the patient by her birth name, Frank. The patient declined my visit. The patient then came to our hospice inpatient unit, and as the RN was helping the patient get settled, the RN asked how the patient wanted to be addressed. The patient said with a sense of resignation and a shrug of the shoulders, "Oh, just do whatever you want." The RN sat next to the patient on the bed, put her arm around the patient's shoulders and said, "I really mean that. How do you want us to talk to you and care for you?" The patient said, "My name is Susan." It is my belief that the RN at our hospice house was the one who provided the spiritual care needed in that moment, and who set the stage for the end-of-life care Susan needed. She died in our Hospice House. Her hair and nails were done, and she was comfortable.

—REV. ANNE G. HUEY, MDIV, MSHS, BCC

Goddess, gods, the Divine, or the Sacred—how are things between you and that power?" Although grammatically awkward, using such inclusive language will communicate to the patients and families you work with that you have an open mind regarding their spiritual, existential, and religious beliefs.

Table 9.3 Spiritual Concerns

Source: Puchalski et al. 2009. Reprinted with permission of Mary Ann Liebert, Inc., © 2009 Mary Ann Liebert, Inc. The publisher for this copyrighted material is Mary Ann Liebert, Inc.

A NOTE ABOUT BEREAVEMENT CARE

After a patient dies, their family of choice, family of origin, or both will likely benefit from bereavement care. Bereavement care should address the psychosocial and spiritual needs of the family and should be delivered in a manner that is sensitive to the unique needs of the individuals. In delivering bereavement care, it is important to remember the historical context of LGBTQ individuals' reluctance to access care and acknowledge the effect that may have on bereavement outcomes. "Those occupying the position of overt exclusion may be at increased risk of adverse bereavement outcomes due to the additional barriers and stressors they experience and, therefore, may need additional support. In addition, for some individuals, due to historical factors, such as having lived through a period when homosexuality was illegal, there may be an expectation of homophobia or assumption of overt exclusion, even if this is not actualized in interactions with healthcare professionals" (Bristowe, Marshall, and Harding 2016).

When recommending a bereavement group to an individual, give careful thought to whether the individual's needs are likely to be met by that particular group. Consider the following factors:

- A man may not feel comfortable in an all-female bereavement group.
- A woman whose female partner just died may feel as though her loss is seen as "less than" the loss experienced by women whose husbands have died.
- A transgender individual in a bereavement group with cisgender persons may feel as though their gender identity and expression is the focal point of the group's attention rather than their experience of grief and loss.
- A bisexual individual may feel as though group members' misconceptions about bisexuality make it difficult for them to recognize the significance of the individual's loss.

- A heterosexual individual may not feel comfortable in a bereavement group comprised entirely of LGB individuals.
- A cisgender individual may not feel comfortable in a bereavement group made up entirely of transgender individuals.
- Heterosexual, cisgender support-group members may not behave in a welcoming way to an LGBTQ person.

In short, every grieving individual is just that—an individual. Never make assumptions about where a person will be most comfortable. Ask questions to determine the bereavement group or groups in which the individual is most likely to feel a sense of safety and support.

KEY POINTS TO REMEMBER

- If a patient or family member appears to be experiencing emotional distress, assess for clinically significant depression and suicidal ideation, document the results of your assessment, and take the appropriate actions, based on your discipline's scope of practice.
- When assessing emotional distress in a patient or family member, be sensitive to the fact that the perceived source of distress could be a long-standing issue that would seem to have nothing to do with the seriousness of the patient's life-limiting illness.
- Don't assume that all lesbian, gay, bisexual, transgender, gender-nonconforming, queer, and/or questioning individuals will be experiencing emotional distress regarding relationships with their family of origin. Many LGBTQ individuals have a positive, supportive relationship with their family of origin.
- Despair, hope, and meaning all play important roles in patients' and families' experiences of growth in the context of advanced illness. It is up to each patient and family to define what hope means for them. Your role is to offer

them information, choices, and support, not permission to hope for a particular outcome.

- There is a difference between a spiritual history and a spiritual assessment. Any member of the team may conduct a spiritual history but only a board-certified chaplain or spiritual-care provider with equivalent training should complete a spiritual assessment.
- When you ask a patient or patient's family about their spiritual/existential needs, the language you use should be neutral, open, and inclusive; they should not be able to guess your own spiritual or religious beliefs based on your questions.
- As you take a patient's spiritual history, remember the mitigation plan discussed in Chapter 1. It is important to prevent your unconscious biases from having a negative impact on the care you provide.
- Spiritual distress may manifest itself in a variety of a ways, many of which may seem to overlap with indicators of psychosocial or emotional distress.
- In delivering bereavement care, it is important to remember the historical context of LGBTQ individuals' reluctance to access care and acknowledge the effect this may have on bereavement outcomes. When recommending a bereavement group to an individual, give careful thought to whether the individual's needs are likely to be met by that particular group.

DISCUSSION QUESTIONS

1. In palliative care and hospice, each member of the interdisciplinary/interprofessional team plays a role in ensuring that the psychosocial needs of patients and families are assessed and addressed. Describe a "psychosocial assessment" and "supportive techniques." What is the role of your discipline in using these tools?

2. What are the similarities and differences between emotional distress and spiritual/existential distress in terms

of presentation and assessment? Which members of the interdisciplinary/interprofessional team address each type of distress?

3. What are the developmental tasks involved in life completion and life closure? What roles do despair, hope, and meaning play in the context of serious and life-threatening illness?

4. Within the context of palliative care and hospice, what is a spiritual/existential assessment and what role, if any, does your discipline play in conducting such an assessment?

5. Describe common experiences of spiritual/existential distress for patients and families facing chronic and life-limiting conditions.

CHAPTER ACTIVITY

Contact a palliative care or hospice chaplain and ask to meet at their workplace for about an hour to learn more about the chaplain's role on the interdisciplinary/interprofessional team. During your meeting, ask the chaplain about spiritual distress and how it presents in palliative care or hospice patients. Ask about the chaplain's experiences working with LGBTQ patients and families and the ways in which the chaplain has supported these patients and families. Afterward, reflect on your meeting. Were you surprised by anything you learned? Do you think working in collaboration with a chaplain would improve the care you deliver to patients in palliative care or hospice? Why or why not?

CHAPTER 10

ENSURING INSTITUTIONAL INCLUSIVENESS

CHAPTER OBJECTIVES

1. Discuss your role in strengthening the inclusion of LGBTQ individuals and families in the palliative care or hospice institution/facility/program in which you work.

2. Assess the inclusiveness of wording on the intake or admission forms your institution/facility/program uses.

3. Assess marketing and outreach materials for inclusive language and imagery.

4. List five policies or benefits that demonstrate an employer's commitment to being LGBTQ-inclusive.

5. List one action you will take in the next month as an individual health care provider to strengthen the inclusion of LGBTQ individuals and their families in your institution/facility/program.

Key Terms: employee benefits, orientation, and training; intake forms and processes; marketing and community engagement

Acquaviva, Kimberly
LGBTQ-Inclusive Hospice and Palliative Care
dx.doi.org/10.17312/harringtonparkpress/2017.03lgbtqihpc.010
© 2017 by Kimberly Acquaviva

The first nine chapters of *LGBTQ-Inclusive Hospice and Palliative Care* describe how individual health care providers can deliver high-quality palliative care and hospice care that is inclusive of LGBTQ individuals and their families. For palliative care and hospice professionals to have the best opportunity to put this knowledge into practice, however, they need to take a few steps at the institutional level to ensure that LGBTQ patients and their families feel welcome and safe coming to them for care. The care that individual health care professionals provide to patients and families is a bit like a clinic on an offshore island. The care provided on that island may be the best in the world, but if patients and families can't reach it, those health care professionals lose out on the opportunity to serve them. This chapter explains how to assess the structural integrity of an institution's bridge to LGBTQ patients, and how to extend and strengthen that bridge to reach, welcome, and serve LGBTQ individuals and their families.

YOUR ROLE IN STRENGTHENING INSTITUTIONAL INCLUSION OF LGBTQ INDIVIDUALS AND FAMILIES

Whether you are an advanced practice registered nurse, physician, registered nurse, chaplain, social worker, or counselor, your profession's code of ethics compels you to advocate for changes at the institutional level to ensure that LGBTQ individuals and their families have access to the same high-quality care available to others:

- **Association of Professional Chaplains**
  "Members shall seek to represent the best interests of those whom they serve[,] giving voice to the vulnerable whenever possible." (Association of Professional Chaplains 2000)

- **National Association of Social Workers**
  "The primary mission of the social work profession is to enhance human well-being and help meet the basic human needs of all people, with particular attention to the needs and

empowerment of people who are vulnerable, oppressed, and living in poverty. . . . Social workers promote social justice and social change with and on behalf of clients. "Clients" is used inclusively to refer to individuals, families, groups, organizations, and communities. Social workers are sensitive to cultural and ethnic diversity and strive to end discrimination, oppression, poverty, and other forms of social injustice. These activities may be in the form of direct practice, community organizing, supervision, consultation administration, advocacy, social and political action, policy development and implementation, education, and research and evaluation. Social workers seek to enhance the capacity of people to address their own needs. Social workers also seek to promote the responsiveness of organizations, communities, and other social institutions to individuals' needs and social problems." (NASW 2008)

- **American Nurses Association**
  "Ethics, human rights, and nursing converge as a formidable instrument for social justice and health diplomacy that can be amplified by collaboration with other health professionals. Nurses understand that the lived experiences of inequality, poverty, and social marginalization contribute to the deterioration of health globally." (ANA 2015)

  "Nurses collaborate with others to change unjust structures and processes that affect both individuals and communities. Structural, social, and institutional inequalities and disparities exacerbate the incidence and burden of illness, trauma, suffering, and premature death." (Ibid.)

  "Nurses must recognize that health care is provided to culturally diverse populations in this country and around the globe. Nurses should collaborate to create a moral milieu that is sensitive to diverse cultural values and practices." (Ibid.)

- **American Medical Association**
  "A physician shall support access to medical care for all people." (AMA 2001)

Each discipline's code of ethics contains language about the importance of advocating for institutional change to ensure access to care, but how do you translate what's written in your discipline's code of ethics into specific actions you can take? If your primary role in your institution involves direct practice with patients and families, you may be unfamiliar or uncomfortable with advocating for institutional-level change. Even the word *advocacy* can sound a bit strident to health care professionals accustomed to focusing on direct patient care in the palliative care and hospice environment. Advocacy does not have to be confrontational, though—in fact, when done well, advocacy feels more collaborative than confrontational to all parties involved. Following are concrete steps you can take within your institution to advocate for greater inclusion of LGBTQ individuals and families.

ASSESSING YOUR BRIDGE TO LGBTQ PATIENTS

As a palliative care or hospice professional, you have an interest in providing LGBTQ-inclusive care. But before LGBTQ individuals and their families can benefit from your knowledge and skills, they need to seek out the services of your program. The bridge between you and potential patients and families is made up of four main "planks," each of which is essential to the structural integrity of the bridge as a mechanism for reaching, welcoming, and serving *all* patients, including LGBTQ individuals and families.

- Plank 1: Nondiscrimination statement
- Plank 2: **Employee benefits, orientation, and training**
- Plank 3: **Intake forms and processes**
- Plank 4: **Marketing and community engagement**

When I speak to hospice and palliative care programs on this topic, participants are often surprised by my heavy focus on employee benefits, policies, orientation, and training. All too often, palliative care and hospice programs approach the challenge of reaching LGBTQ individuals and their families primarily through marketing. Although marketing is an important plank in the bridge to LGBTQ people and their families, the bridge won't be strong enough unless the other planks are in place.

PLANK 1: NONDISCRIMINATION STATEMENT

Of all the planks in your program's bridge, your organization's nondiscrimination statement is the most important. Your nondiscrimination statement needs to be two things — inclusive and visible — if it is going to be an effective tool for reaching and welcoming LGBTQ individuals and their families.

An LGBTQ-inclusive nondiscrimination statement will include the phrases "gender identity," "gender expression," and "sexual orientation" in addition to the other phrases that commonly appear in nondiscrimination statements. It's not enough to list "sex" and "sexual orientation" — the statement needs to be specific in conveying a commitment not to discriminate against transgender individuals. Lambda Legal recommends an even broader and more inclusive approach, and urges organizations to "establish nondiscrimination, fair visitation[,] and other policies that prohibit bias and discrimination based on sexual orientation, gender identity and expression[,] and HIV status, recognize families of LGBTQ people and their wishes[,] and provide a process for reporting and redressing discrimination if it occurs" (Lambda Legal 2010).

Imagine that you are a transgender individual trying to choose a palliative care or hospice program. What would you think about the following nondiscrimination statements (based on actual statements found online) and how would they make you feel? What about if you were bisexual? Gay or lesbian?

- **Statement 1:** It is the policy of _____ that no person shall, on the grounds of race, color, national origin, ancestry, age (over 40), sex, genetic information, handicap or disability (including AIDS, HIV infection, or AIDS-related condition), or religious creed, be excluded from participation in, be denied benefits of, or otherwise be subject to discrimination or harassment in the provision of any care or service or employment.

- **Statement 2:** No person shall be discriminated against based on the grounds of race, color, religion, age, sex, sexual orientation, gender identity, national origin, ancestry, marital status, protected veteran status, pregnancy, or disability, or any other categories protected by federal or state law.

- **Statement 3:** _____ does not discriminate against any person on the basis of race, color, creed, national origin, gender, age, sexual orientation, religion, veteran status, or disability.

- **Statement 4:** _____ is committed to a policy of non-discrimination for patients, employees, and visitors. No person shall be subjected to discrimination in the provision of any care or service on the grounds of race, color, national origin (including limited English proficiency), ancestry, age, sex, religion, handicap, disability, or other legally protected basis. Applicants for staff positions shall not be denied membership or particular privileges/ duties on the basis of race, color, national origin (including limited English proficiency), ancestry, religion, or sex.

- **Statement 5:** Patient services are provided without regard to race, religion, age, gender, gender identity, gender expression, sexual orientation, mental or physical disability, communicable disease, or place of national origin.

- **Statement 6:** We care for all people regardless of ability to pay, race, disability, color, creed, religion, gender, age, sexual orientation, gender expression, national origin, ancestry, citizenship, or veteran status.

The variability in the wording of these nondiscrimination statements is striking. How do you think _your_ organization's nondiscrimination statement should read? Your organization should revise its nondiscrimination statement until you can answer yes to all of the following questions:

- Does the statement include all language required under the Federal Civil Rights Act of 1964?
- Does the statement include all language required under the Equal Pay Act of 1963?
- Does the statement include all language required under the Age Discrimination in Employment Act of 1967?
- Does the statement include all language required under the Rehabilitation Act of 1973?
- Does the statement include all language required under the Americans with Disabilities Act of 1991?
- Does the statement include all language required under other federal labor and employment laws?
- Does the statement include all language required under your state's human relations, labor, and employment laws?
- Does the statement include all language required under your city's human relations, labor, and employment laws?
- Does the statement include the phrases "sexual orientation," "gender identity," and "gender expression"?

It is important to point out that if your organization is not formally committed to a policy of nondiscrimination based on sexual orientation, gender identity, and gender expression or gender presentation in its employment practices, you should not expect lesbian, gay, bisexual, transgender, gender-nonconforming, queer, and/or questioning patients and families to feel safe seeking out your services.

Your organization's nondiscrimination statement should be a highly visible manifestation of its commitment to inclusion. Unfortunately, many palliative care and hospice programs have nondiscrimination statements that are, at best, difficult to find online and, at worst, completely absent from the organization's website. So how should your organization disseminate its nondiscrimination statement? When the nondiscrimination statement is put forth correctly, your organization should be able to answer yes to all of the following questions:

- Is the nondiscrimination statement on the organization's home page online (not buried somewhere else on the website)?
- When a visitor to the organization's website types the term *gay, lesbian, bisexual, transgender, discrimination, gender identity, gender expression,* or *sexual orientation* into any search boxes embedded on your website, does the search yield a link to the nondiscrimination statement?
- When someone enters the name of your organization and the word *discrimination* in the Google search box, does the search yield a link to your organization's nondiscrimination statement?
- Is your organization's nondiscrimination statement included on *every* brochure and flyer?
- If someone calls your organization's main phone number and asks about your nondiscrimination policy, will the caller be read the nondiscrimination statement directly, *without being transferred to someone else?*
- When someone asks *you* what the organization's nondiscrimination policy is, do you know what to say?

If aspects of your organization's nondiscrimination statement need to be revised or strengthened, set up a meeting with the most senior administrator you have access to and say you wish to discuss an easy, low-cost way the organization can attract and serve more people in the community. When you pitch the nondiscrimination policy as a way to increase patient access and enrollment at little cost to the organization, you may stand a greater chance of getting that meeting.

It can take years of gentle but persistent advocacy to get an organization to change its nondiscrimination statement, so don't give up. Your persistence, politeness, and professionalism will go a long way toward transforming your organization into one that clearly articulates its commitment to inclusion and nondiscrimination. Once your organization's nondiscrimination statement is both inclusive and visible, you will be ready to move on to strengthening and extending other aspects of your bridge to LGBTQ individuals and their families.

PLANK 2: EMPLOYEE BENEFITS, ORIENTATION, AND TRAINING

For your organization to be a place where LGBTQ individuals and their families feel safe and comfortable accessing services, it needs to be a place where LGBTQ employees feel safe, comfortable, and valued. If your organization can answer yes to all of the following questions, this plank is likely to be a strong part of your bridge to LGBTQ individuals and their families.

- Is there parity "between employees with different-sex spouses and same sex partners or spouses in the provision of the following benefits: COBRA; dental; vision; legal dependent coverage; bereavement leave; employer-provided supplemental life insurance for a partner; relocation/travel assistance; adoption assistance; qualified joint and survivor annuity for partners; qualified pre-retirement survivor annuity for partners; retiree healthcare benefits; and employee discounts" (Human Rights Campaign Foundation 2016)?
- Does your organization offer "equal health coverage for transgender individuals without exclusion for medically necessary care"(ibid.)?
- Does your organization have "gender transition guidelines with supportive restroom, dress code[,] and documentation guidance" (ibid.)?
- Does your organization include optional questions on sexual orientation and gender identity on its employee data collection forms?
- Does your organization currently have any gay, lesbian, bisexual, or transgender employees? Are there any gay, lesbian, bisexual, or transgender employees in management or leadership positions?

- Do the orientation and training materials for new employees include the nondiscrimination policy?
- Does your organization "require health profession students and health professionals to undergo significant cultural competency training about sexual orientation, gender identity[,] and expression" (Lambda Legal 2010)?
- Does your organization's new-employee orientation "include training about the specific ways LGBTQ people and people living with HIV who are also people of color, low income, seniors[,] or members of other underserved populations may experience discrimination in health care settings and establish policies to prevent them" (ibid.)?

Convincing your organization to be inclusive in its approach to employee benefits, orientation, and training may seem like a steep hill to climb, given concerns about potential cost, but in reality the steepest climb is getting an inclusive non-discrimination statement. After that, employee policies fall into place more easily. Once the first two planks of your organization's bridge to LGBTQ individuals and their families are in place, you are ready to focus on intake processes.

PLANK 3: INTAKE FORMS AND PROCESSES

When a potential patient or family member contacts your organization, the first interaction they have with an employee or volunteer can have a profound effect on whether they feel welcome and safe in seeking your organization's services. Think about who those crucial first points of contact are in your organization. They might be phone or switchboard operators, website administrators, social media directors, administrative assistants, members of the admissions team, volunteers, or all of the above. If a potential client called any of the people in these positions and asked whether your organization has the training and experience needed to care for a bisexual patient, for example, what would they be told? What if someone called and asked, "Are you comfortable taking care of gay patients?" or "Has your program ever cared for a transgender woman?" If you are not sure how your organization's gatekeepers would answer, have a friend call and ask some of these questions. I am a big fan of the "mystery shopper" approach when it comes to getting an accurate sense of what patients and families experience when they call an organization. Every employee in your organization who is a potential first point of contact with the public should be taught how to answer such questions warmly and accurately.

When patients are in the process of being admitted to your program or service, you have an opportunity to communicate your commitment to honoring their values, customs, and preferences. Thus the intake forms your organization uses need to be inclusive. Consider incorporating the following questions on the forms and in the intake process:

- What name would you like to be called?
- What gender pronouns do you go by (e.g., he/him, she/her, them/their, ze/zir)?
- What sex were you assigned at birth?
- What gender do you identify as now?
- What word or words would you use to describe your sexual orientation?

Once your organization has revised its nondiscrimination statement; strengthened its employee benefits, orientation, and training; and revised its intake forms and processes, it will be ready to begin marketing its services to LGBTQ individuals and their families.

PLANK 4: MARKETING AND COMMUNITY ENGAGEMENT

With your organizational house in order, it's time to reach out directly, through marketing and community engagement, to welcome LGBTQ individuals and their families. Interestingly, if your organization has put the first three planks of the bridge to LGBTQ patients and their families in place, it won't need to spend much money on marketing. A visible commitment to equality, inclusion, and nondiscrimination will yield tremendous word-of-mouth benefits.

Let's start by taking a look at your marketing materials. If your only data sources were the photographs on your organization's website and brochures, what would you conclude about the types of people your organization serves? Would gay, lesbian, bisexual, or transgender individuals see themselves reflected in the images they see? Do any of the images show same-gender dyads, or are they all photos of male-female couples? Are all the people in the images white? Do the photos depicting patient or staff diversity appear awkward or forced? (My personal pet peeve: photographs that seem like crayon-box lineups: one person of each race, gender, age, and so on). Your organization's website and brochures should feature images that reflect the communities you already serve *and* the communities you are striving to serve.

Where does your organization spend its advertising and outreach dollars? If you are not doing so already, you may want to consider advertising in a local LGBTQ newspaper. Putting up an information booth at an LGBTQ pride festival can help to familiarize members of the community with your organization and the services it offers. Your organization could also offer an LGBTQ-specific bereavement group as a community engagement tool.

WHAT NOW?

The path to creating and sustaining an LGBTQ-inclusive palliative care or hospice program is not a linear one with a clear beginning and end. The journey requires an ongoing commitment to reassessing and strengthening your organization's policies, programs, services, and outreach efforts, and as such, it's an iterative process in which your organization will continually be engaged. You have the knowledge and skills to be a catalyst for change, and in reading this book you have demonstrated a commitment to providing LGBTQ-inclusive palliative and hospice care. So what are you going to do to strengthen the inclusion of LGBTQ individuals and their families at your workplace? Decide on one action you will take in the next month, write it down, and make it happen.

KEY POINTS TO REMEMBER

- Whether you are an APRN, physician, RN, chaplain, social worker, or counselor, your profession's code of ethics compels you to advocate for changes at the institutional level to ensure that LGBTQ individuals and families have access to the same high-quality care available to others.
- The bridge between you and potential patients and families is made up of four main planks, each of which is essential to the structural integrity of the bridge as a mechanism for reaching, welcoming, and serving LGBTQ individuals and families.

    Plank 1: Nondiscrimination statement
    Plank 2: Employee benefits, orientation, and training
    Plank 3: Intake forms and processes
    Plank 4: Marketing and community engagement
- Your organization's nondiscrimination statement needs to be two things—inclusive and visible—if it is going to be an effective tool for reaching and welcoming LGBTQ individuals and their families.
- An inclusive nondiscrimination statement is one that includes the phrases "gender identity," "gender expression," and "sexual orientation," in addition to the other phrases that commonly appear in nondiscrimination statements.
- If your organization is not formally committed to a policy of nondiscrimination based on sexual orientation, gender identity, and gender expression or gender presentation in its employment practices, you should not expect lesbian, gay, bisexual, transgender, gender-nonconforming, queer, and/or questioning patients and families to feel safe seeking out your services.

- Your organization's nondiscrimination statement should be a highly visible manifestation of its commitment to inclusion.
- For your organization to be a place where LGBTQ individuals and their families feel safe and comfortable receiving services, it needs to be a place where LGBTQ employees feel safe, comfortable, and valued.
- When patients are being admitted to your program or service, you have an opportunity to communicate your commitment to honoring their values, customs, and preferences. Thus the intake forms and processes used by your organization need to be inclusive.
- A visible commitment to equality, inclusion, and non-discrimination will yield tremendous word-of-mouth benefits.
- Make sure your website, brochures, and other marketing materials depict images inclusive of LGBTQ individuals and families.

DISCUSSION QUESTIONS

1. Can individual palliative care or hospice professionals improve the inclusion of LGBTQ patients and families in the programs where they work? Why or why not? Do individual professionals have an ethical obligation to advocate for institutional change in order to facilitate the inclusion of LGBTQ individuals and families? Why or why not?

2. Describe five policies and/or employee benefits that demonstrate an employer's commitment to being LGBTQ-inclusive. How do inclusive policies and employee benefits strengthen the inclusion of LGBTQ patients and families?

3. What does the wording on your program's intake or admission forms (or those of a program in your community) say about the program's commitment to recognizing and serving LGBTQ patients and families? What changes could be made to the wording to make it more inclusive?

4. What do the wording and imagery on your program's website and brochures (or those of a program in your community) say about the program's commitment to recognizing and serving LGBTQ patients and families? What changes could be made to the wording and imagery to make them more inclusive?

5. Describe one action you will take in the next month as an individual health care provider to strengthen the inclusion of LGBTQ individuals and their families in your program (or in a program in your community).

CHAPTER ACTIVITY

List at least ten actions your program or organization could take to improve its inclusion of LGBTQ patients and families. Share your list of recommendations with someone who has the power to implement them, and then ask them what you can do to help with the implementation process.

GLOSSARY

access to care Availability of care and "the timely use of personal health services to achieve the best health outcomes" (IOM 1993).

advance care planning The process of "making plans for the health care [a patient wants] during a serious illness" (Administration for Community Living n.d.). Advance care planning as facilitated by palliative care and hospice professionals entails four core components: (1) educating patients about their illness; (2) providing patients with information about treatment options, benefits, and burden; (3) facilitating discussions between patients and families regarding treatment options, preferences, and decisions; and (4) assisting patients in documenting their preferences and decisions in writing.

advance directive "A general term that describes two types of legal documents: (1) Living will, and (2) Healthcare power of attorney. These documents allow [patients] to instruct others about [their] future healthcare wishes and appoint a person to make healthcare decisions if [they] are not able to speak for [themselves]" (National Hospice and Palliative Care Organization 2016).

affirmation Acknowledging the accuracy of a patient's statement or encouraging patients' efforts to make sense of their experience.

anger "A strong feeling of annoyance, displeasure, antagonism, irritation, or rage" (Gladding 2011).

anxiety "The apprehensive anticipation of future danger or misfortune accompanied by a feeling of worry, distress, and/or somatic symptoms of tension. The focus of anticipated danger may be internal or external" (American Psychiatric Association 2013b).

asexual Some individuals do not identify as having sexual, emotional, or relational attractions to anyone. These individuals may refer to themselves as asexual.

assumption "A willingness to accept something as true without question or proof" (*Cambridge Dictionary Online* n.d.).

attitude "A relatively stable and enduring predisposition to respond positively or negatively to a person, object, situation, institution, or event. An attitude carries a strong emotional component; when generalized, it becomes a stereotype" (Gladding 2011).

autonomy One of the four ethical principles specifying the duties of health care professionals to their patients. Autonomy refers to patients' right to make choices for themselves so long as they have the capacity to make those choices (Beauchamp and Childress 2013).

barriers to care Factors that make it difficult for LGBTQ individuals to seek and/or accept hospice and palliative care. Barriers to care generally fall into three categories: **financial barri-**

ers to care, institutional barriers to care, and **perceptual barriers to care.**

belief "Conviction of the truth of some statement or the reality of some being or phenomenon especially when based on examination of evidence" (*Merriam-Webster Dictionary* 2015).

beneficence One of the four ethical principles specifying the duties of health care professionals to their patients. Beneficence means "to help the patient advance his/her own good" (Vermont Ethics Network 2011b) or to help the patient benefit, as defined by that patient (Beauchamp and Childress 2013).

bereavement "The state of having lost through death someone with whom one has had a close relationship. This state includes a range of grief and mourning responses" (American Psychiatric Association 2013b).

bisexual Having a sexual orientation or attraction toward both sexes. A person who is bisexual is attracted to both men and women; commonly referred to as "bi."

breathlessness (or *shortness of breath, dyspnea*) "Few sensations are as frightening as not being able to get enough air. Although shortness of breath — known medically as dyspnea — is likely to be experienced differently by different people, it's often described as an intense tightening in the chest or feeling of suffocation" (Mayo Foundation for Medical Education and Research n.d.a).

CAMPERS A mnemonic device developed by the author to facilitate greater self-awareness among providers. The letters stand for clear purpose, attitudes and beliefs, mitigation plan, patient, emotions, reactions, and strategy.

care coordination "An approach in which all members of the [interdisciplinary] team work together to plan for a patient's care" (Center to Advance Palliative Care 2012a).

chosen family See **family of choice.**

clinical note "A notation of a contact with the patient and/or the family that is written and dated by any person providing services and that describes signs and symptoms, treatments and medications administered, including the patient's reaction and/or response, and any changes in physical, emotional, psychosocial or spiritual condition during a given period of time" (CMS 2015b).

compassion "A response to the perceived suffering of others that requires listening intently and acting in a concerned, kind, and empathic way" (Gladding 2011).

competence "Competence is a legal term that is determined by a judge, and it is typically an all-or-nothing assessment. In other words, a patient is either competent or incompetent. . . . Decision-making capacity [DMC], on the other hand, is a clinical determination made by a medical professional. . . . DMC is decision-dependent, meaning that a patient might have sufficient DMC to make a relatively straightforward decision, but not enough to make a complex medical decision. . . . In general, higher levels of DMC are required for decisions that are complex, have potentially grave consequences, or when a patient is making a decision contrary to what most people would opt for" (Vermont Ethics Network 2011a).

comprehensive assessment In the hospice context, "a thorough evaluation of the patient's physical, psychosocial, emotional and spiritual status related to the terminal illness and related conditions. This includes a thorough evaluation of the caregiver's and family's willingness and capability to care for the patient" (CMS 2015b).

comprehensive history A complete history that generally includes the patient's birth sex and true gender identity; the patient's understanding of his or her illness and prognosis; information about the patient's advance directives; the patient's goals for care; a history of the patient's illness and physical symptoms; a psychosocial history and spiritual history; the patient's sexual orientation and sexual behavior; a surgical history; an assessment of the patient's activities of daily living; an assessment of the patient's quality of life; a depression screening; a list of pharmacologic, nonpharmacologic, and complementary/alternative therapies; a list of allergies and drug interactions; and information regarding substance abuse or dependency. In palliative care and hospice care, the **Five-Dimension Assessment Model** provides a framework for taking a comprehensive history.

confidentiality "The obligation of confidentiality prohibits the health care provider from disclosing information about the patient's case to others without permission and encourages the providers and health care systems to take precautions to ensure that only authorized access occurs" (De Bord, Burke, and Dudzinski 2013).

confusion (also *disorientation*) When a patient cannot remember or is unclear "about the time of day, date, or season (time); where one is (place); or who one is (person)" (American Psychiatric Association 2013b).

constipation "A condition in which bowel movements are infrequent or incomplete" (*Stedman's Medical Dictionary* 2006).

coping skills "The skills and behaviors people use to adjust to their environments and avoid stress" (Gladding 2011).

DAROP format A psychosocial documentation format developed by Russell Hilliard, DAROP stands for data, action, results, observations, and plan.

decision-making capacity "Patients with decision-making capacity (DMC) have the right to refuse any treatment, even one that is life-sustaining. They also have the right to choose between treatment options, based on the principle of informed consent. Generally only when a patient lacks DMC does their Advance Directive or **health care proxy** have a role in medical decision-making.

For these reasons it's very important to determine whether a patient has DMC, which sometimes is a difficult determination to make, especially in cases of delirium or progressive dementia. . . . DMC is not the same as 'competence'" (Vermont Ethics Network 2011a).

denial "A defense mechanism in which a person ignores or disavows unacceptable thoughts or acts as if an experience does not exist or never did" (Gladding 2011).

depression A general term used to describe a variety of depressive disorders: "disruptive mood dysregulation disorder, major depressive disorder (including major depressive episode), persistent depressive disorder (dysthymia), premenstrual dysphoric disorder, substance/medication-induced depressive disorder, depressive disorder due to another medical condition, other specified depressive disorder, and unspecified depressive disorder. . . . The common feature of all of these disorders is the presence of sad, empty, or irritable mood, accompanied by somatic and cognitive changes that significantly affect the individual's capacity to function. What differs among them are issues of duration, timing, or presumed etiology" (American Psychiatric Association 2013b).

despair "An inability . . . to find meaning in one's life. . . . A complete loss of hope" (Gladding 2011).

disposal of supplies Supplies such as used syringes and lancets, soiled incontinence pads, and used gauze and bandages must be disposed of safely and effectively; refers to the skills that patients and their caregivers require to carry this out.

do-not-resuscitate order (also *do-not-attempt-resuscitation order* and *allow-natural-death order* "A do-not-resuscitate order, or DNR order, is a medical order written by a doctor. It instructs health care providers not to do cardiopulmonary resuscitation (CPR) if a patient's breathing stops or if the patient's heart stops beating. A DNR order allows you to choose whether or not you want CPR[,] before an emergency occurs. It is specific about CPR. It does not provide instructions for other treatments, such as pain medicine, other medicines, or nutrition. The doctor writes the order only after talking about it with the patient (if possible), the proxy, or the patient's family" (National Library of Medicine 2016).

durable power of attorney for health care See health care power of attorney.

emotion "A strong feeling or affect of any kind. . . . The so-called Big Four feelings . . . are anger, sadness, fear, and joy" (Gladding 2011).

emotional distress "An emotional . . . state of pain, sorrow, misery, suffering, or discomfort" (*Mosby's Medical Dictionary* 2009). Sometimes referred to as psychological distress.

empathic behaviors Things caregivers say or do to convey to patients that they care about them and are committed to understanding their perspectives or experiences.

empathy "The [health care provider's] ability to see, be aware of, conceptualize, understand, and effectively communicate back to a [patient] the [patient's] feelings, thoughts, and frame of reference in regard to a situation or points of view" (Gladding 2011). (Note: I have replaced Gladding's terms *counselor* and *client* with the terms *health care provider* and *patient*.)

employee benefits, orientation, and training The ways in which an organization orients, trains, and supports its employees, ideally in a manner consistent with the organization's mission, vision, and values.

employment discrimination Consists of "bias in hiring, promotion, job assignment, termination, compensation, retaliation, and various types of harassment" (Legal Information Institute n.d.).

end-stage disease "A disease condition that is essentially terminal because of irreversible damage to vital tissues or organs" (*Mosby's Medical Dictionary* 2009).

end-stage disease progression clinical status, symptoms, and other signs and indicators suggestive of progression of end-stage disease.

environmental and safety assessment An assessment undertaken of the patient's living environment to prevent accidents and falls and to facilitate the continued independence of the patient.

ethical principles "In the U.S., four main principles define the ethical duties that health care professionals owe to patients. They are: **Autonomy**: to honor the patient's right to make their own decision; **Beneficence**: to help the patient advance his/her own good; **Nonmaleficence**: to do no harm; and **Justice**: to be fair and treat like cases alike" (Vermont Ethics Network 2011b).

expected outcomes Outcomes that align with stated goals of care. A statement of expected outcome will contain a subject ("Mr. Jones"), a verb in future tense ("will sleep"), a condition ("without a sleeping pill"), a criterion ("for at least 4 consecutive hours"), and a time ("tonight"): Mr. Jones will sleep without a sleeping pill for at least 4 consecutive hours tonight.

eye contact "Looking at someone in the eye when interviewing them" (Gladding 2011).

eye-level approach Entering into an interaction with a patient in a manner that ensures the caregiver's eyes are level with those of the patient. For example, if a patient is in bed, you would pull up a chair and sit next to the bed so that your eyes were as close to level as possible with those of the patient. This helps to minimize the power imbalance between provider and patient and facilitates rapport.

facilitating behaviors The things said or done to foster open communication with a patient.

family of choice (also *chosen family*) The "persons or group of people an individual sees as significant in their life. It may include none, all, or some members of their family of origin. In addition, it may include individuals such as significant others, domestic partners, friends, and coworkers" (Gender Equity Resource Center 2013).

family of origin The family (by birth, adoption, or informal kinship care) in which a person was raised as a child.

fatigue "A state (also called exhaustion, tiredness, lethargy, languidness, languor, lassitude, and listlessness) usually associated with a weakening or depletion of one's physical and/or mental resources, ranging from a general state of lethargy to a specific, work-induced burning sensation within one's muscles. Physical fatigue leads to an inability to continue functioning at one's normal level of activity. Although widespread in everyday life, this state usually becomes particularly noticeable during heavy exercise. Mental fatigue, by contrast, most often manifests as somnolence (sleepiness)" (American Psychiatric Association 2013b).

fear "An emotional response to perceived imminent threat or danger associated with urges to flee or fight" (American Psychiatric Association 2013b).

FICA Spiritual History Tool Developed by Christina Puchalski, the FICA Spiritual History Tool © is a widely used tool for assessing and addressing spiritual issues with patients. FICA stands for faith or belief, importance, community, and address in care (Puchalski 1996).

financial barriers to care Financial concerns (actual or perceived) regarding the degree to which an individual can afford to receive palliative care or hospice care.

Five-Dimension Assessment Model A practical framework for taking a comprehensive history of patients in palliative care and hospice care. The Five-Dimension Assessment Model incorporates questions about birth sex, gender identity, sexual orientation, sexual behavior, and sexual health into the assessment process and places the primary focus on the "patient as person." The five dimensions in the model are: Patient as Person (Part 1); Illness/Treatment Summary; Functional Activities and Symptoms; Decision-Making; Anticipatory Planning for Death; and Patient as Person (Part 2). The model, developed by the author, is based on a synthesis of the extant literature on patient and family assessment in palliative and hospice care.

focused history (also *history of present illness*) A patient history narrowly focused on the presenting symptom, problem, or illness.

gender "The public (and usually legally recognized) lived role as boy or girl, man or woman. Biological factors are seen as contributing in interaction with social and psychological factors to gender development" (American Psychiatric Association 2013b).

gender-affirmation surgery (also *sex reassignment surgery*) "Surgery to change primary and/or secondary sex characteristics to affirm a person's gender identity. Sex reassignment surgery can be an important part of medically necessary treatment to alleviate gender dysphoria" (World Professional Association for Transgender Health 2012).

gender discordance When a person's anatomical/biological sex and gender identity do not match (Adelson and Bockting 2014).

gender dysphoria "Distress that accompanies the incongruence between one's experienced and expressed gender and one's assigned or natal gender" (American Psychiatric Association 2013b).

gender expression The way individuals express or present to others their internal sense of masculinity or femininity. Also called **gender presentation.**

gender identity "A category of social identity that refers to an individual's identification as male, female or . . . some category other than male or female" (American Psychiatric Association 2013b).

gender nonconformity A term that describes behavior (including appearance and dress) that fails to conform to socially constructed norms or expectations for a given gender (Adelson and Bockting 2014).

gender presentation See **gender expression.**

genderqueer "A person whose gender identity and/or gender expression falls outside of the dominant societal norm for their assigned sex, is beyond genders, or is some combination of them" (University of California, Davis 2015).

gender reassignment "A change of gender that can be either medical (hormones, surgery) or legal (government recognition), or both. In case of medical interventions, often referred to as *sex reassignment*" (American Psychiatric Association 2013b).

genogram A diagram that shows the emotional relationships between individuals in a family.

goals of care "The goals of care are determined by a patient's priorities and values, their hopes and fears. Goals can be described in plain language without reference to procedures or medical interventions. Possible goals include wanting to live independently, to be able to read books, to play with one's grandchildren, to recognize the people one loves, or simply to live as long as possible. Goals often change over time and should be revisited regularly with one's [clinicians] and loved ones" (Vermont Ethics Network 2011c).

grief "An intense emotional response to a loss characterized by sorrow and distress" (Gladding 2011).

guilt "An emotional response to having done something wrong or having failed to do something" (Gladding 2011).

health care ethics "Health care ethics (a/k/a 'medical' ethics or 'bioethics'), at its simplest, is a set of moral principles, beliefs and values that guide us in making choices about medical care. At the core of health care ethics is our sense of right and wrong and our beliefs about rights we possess and duties we owe others. . . . All 4 principles are considered to be in effect at all times. In theory, each is of equal weight or importance. In practice, however, at least in the US, respect for patient autonomy often takes priority over the others" (Vermont Ethics Network 2011b).

health care power of attorney (also *durable power of attorney for health care*) "A healthcare power of attorney . . . permits the appointed person to make medical decisions for [the patient] if [the patient] cannot make those decisions [him- or herself]. It does not authorize the person to handle . . . financial affairs, and normally does not empower him or her to make decisions while [the patient] can still make them. . . . Most healthcare powers of attorney go into effect when [the patient's] physician concludes that [the patient is] unable to make [his or her] own decisions. If [the patient] regain[s] the ability to make decisions, [the] agent cannot continue to act for [him or her]. Many states have additional requirements that apply only to decisions about life-sustaining medical treatments" (National Hospice and Palliative Care Organization 2016).

health care proxy "Similar to a durable power of attorney for healthcare: a document that designates the person you trust to make medical decisions on your behalf if you are unable" (Center to Advance Palliative Care 2012a).

heterosexual A heterosexual woman is primarily attracted to men and a heterosexual man is primarily attracted to women; both are commonly referred to as "straight."

homosexual A man whose sexual orientation is homosexual (a man who is "gay") is primarily attracted to men. A woman whose sexual orientation is homosexual (who is "lesbian" or "gay") is primarily attracted to women.

hope "The belief that what is desired is also possible and that events will turn out for the best . . . [and] the feeling that what one believes will occur" (Gladding 2011).

hospice "Considered a model of quality care, hospice focuses on relieving symptoms and supporting patients with a life expectancy of months, not years. Hospice involves a team-oriented approach to expert medical care, pain management and emotional and spiritual support. The emphasis is on caring, not curing. In most cases hospice care is provided to a patient in his or her own home. It also can be provided in freestanding hospice facilities, hospitals, nursing homes and other long-term care facilities" (Center to Advance Palliative Care 2012a). "Hospice care means a comprehensive set of services described in Section 1861(dd)(1) of the Act, identified and coordinated by an interdisciplinary group (IDG) to provide for the physical, psychosocial, spiritual, and emotional needs of a terminally ill patient and/or family members, as delineated in a specific patient plan of care" (CMS 2015b).

housing discrimination Discriminatory practices that interfere with an individual's ability to rent or purchase housing.

humor "The ability to laugh at oneself and one's circumstances in a healthy, therapeutic, and nondefensive way" (Gladding 2011).

informed consent "The process by which a patient learns about and understands the purpose, benefits, and potential risks of a medical or surgical intervention, including clinical trials, and then agrees to receive the treatment or participate in the trial. Informed consent generally requires the patient or responsible party to sign a statement confirming that they understand the risks and benefits of the procedure or treatment" (MedicineNet 2012).

insomnia "Inability to sleep, in the absence of external impediments (noise, a bright light) during the period when sleep should normally occur; may vary in degree from restlessness or disturbed slumber to a curtailment of the normal length of sleep or to absolute wakefulness" (*Stedman's Medical Dictionary* 2006).

institutional barriers to care Barriers erected (often unintentionally) by palliative care and hospice care programs that prevent LGBTQ individuals and their families from accessing services. Institutional barriers may include: discriminatory admission and/or employment policies; lack of marketing and outreach materials; and lack of or inadequate orientation and training for health care providers, staff, and volunteers.

intake forms and processes The human, electronic, and paper mechanisms by which an organization or program communicates a sense of welcoming, safety, and inclusion to new patients and families. Includes both "official" mechanisms like admissions processes and forms, and "unofficial" mechanism like interactions with phone or switchboard operators, administrative assistants, volunteers, and so on. When official mechanisms like intake forms are not LGBTQ-inclusive, LGBTQ patients and families may be reluctant to seek or accept services.

interdisciplinary/interprofessional team In the context of hospice care, the team generally consists of "the patient's personal physician; Hospice physician (or medical director); Nurses; Home health aides; Social workers; Clergy or other counselors; Trained volunteers; and Speech, physical, and occupational therapists, if needed" (National Hospice and Palliative Care Organization 2015a). In the context of palliative care, the team generally consists of "palliative care doctors, nurses and social workers. . . . [M]assage therapists, pharmacists, nutritionists and others might also be part of the team" (Center to Advance Palliative Care 2012b).

justice One of the four ethical principles specifying the duties of health care professionals to their patients. Refers to treating patients in a fair and equitable way (Beauchamp and Childress 2013).

lesbian A woman whose sexual orientation is homosexual ("lesbian" or "gay") and who is primarily attracted to women.

life completion and life closure The facilitation of ongoing personal growth and fulfillment throughout the remainder of a person's life. Byock's "developmental taskwork" provides a clearly articulated model for the developmental tasks associated with life completion and life closure (see Byock 1994).

life review "The review of one's life . . . to find themes, meaning, understanding, and acceptance of what one has done" (Gladding 2011).

listening "Listening involves hearing not only the content of a [patient's] words but also the tone and inflection of what is being said" (Gladding 2011). (Note: I have replaced Gladding's term *client's* with *patient's*.)

living will "A written or video statement about the kind of medical care a person does or does not want under certain specific conditions"; designed for use when or if the person is unable to express those wishes (Institute of Medicine 2015).

marketing and community engagement The ways in which an organization or program promotes its services (through marketing) and engages in mutually beneficial relationships with people and entities in the community (via community engagement).

meaning A sense of "having significance and purposefulness" (Gladding 2011).

medication management The skills needed by a patient and/or caregiver to store, organize, administer, and discard the patient's medications safely and effectively.

medication reconciliation Involves "creating the most accurate list possible of all medications a patient is taking—including drug name, dosage, frequency, and route—and comparing that list against the [clinician's] admission, transfer, and/or discharge orders, with the goal of providing correct medications to the patient at all transition points" (Institute for Healthcare Improvement 2016). For a detailed guide to medication reconciliation, see *Medications at Transitions and Clinical Handoffs (MATCH) Toolkit for Medication Reconciliation* (Gleason et al. 2012).

nausea/vomiting "Nausea is feeling an urge to vomit. It is often called 'being sick to your stomach.' Vomiting or throwing-up is forcing the contents of the stomach up through the esophagus and out of the mouth" (National Library of Medicine 2015b).

nonverbal communication "The use of nonverbal behaviors such as eye contact, body position, and physical distance in building a . . . relationship" (Gladding 2011).

nonmaleficence One of the four ethical principles specifying the duties of health care professionals to their patients. Nonmaleficence means to do no harm (Beauchamp and Childress 2013).

normalization Conveying to patients that "they are not alone in their difficulty (e.g., [that] most people have experienced mild depression in the course of their lives)" (Gladding 2011).

open posture "Positioning the body with the torso leaning toward the person being addressed, the arms at one's sides, and the chest, abdomen, and lower extremities easily seen. This form of body positioning during communication implies that one is actively listening and emotionally available to the client or patient. By contrast, a closed posture (in which one leans back, crosses one's arms on the chest and crosses the legs) implies that a person is less receptive to the other person" (*Medical Dictionary* 2009).

out-of-hospital/provider/physician/ medical order for life-sustaining treatment (POLST/MOLST) A document that varies from state to state in format, name, and powers, but that in general "provides medical orders for current treatment" for "persons with serious illness" (National POLST Paradigm 2015).

pain "An unpleasant sensory and emotional experience associated with actual or potential tissue damage, or described in terms of such damage. Note: The inability to communicate verbally does not negate the possibility that an individual is experiencing pain and is in need of appropriate pain-relieving treatment. Pain is always subjective. . . . Many people report pain in the absence of tissue damage or any likely pathophysiological cause; usually this happens for psychological reasons. . . . If they regard their experience as pain, and if they report it in the same ways as pain caused by tissue damage, it should be accepted as pain. This definition avoids tying pain to the stimulus" (International Association for the Study of Pain 2012).

pain and symptom management The process of assessing and addressing symptoms including but not limited to anxiety, breathlessness, confusion, constipation, depression, insomnia, nausea/vomiting, pain, weakness/ fatigue, and weight loss. Patients and families can be taught skills to manage pain and other symptoms at home.

pain management The use of "pharmacological, nonpharmacological, and other approaches to prevent, reduce, or stop pain sensations" (*Gale Encyclopedia of Medicine* 2008).

palliative care "Palliative care means patient- and family-centered care that optimizes quality of life by anticipating, preventing, and treating suffering. Palliative care throughout the continuum of illness involves addressing physical, intellectual, emotional, social, and spiritual needs and [facilitating] patient autonomy, access to information, and choice" (CMS 2015b).

palliative sedation "The intentional lowering of awareness towards, and including, unconsciousness for patients with severe and refractory symptoms" (AAHPM 2014). Also defined as "the use of specific sedative medications to relieve intolerable suffering from refractory symptoms by a reduction in patient consciousness, using appropriate drugs carefully titrated to the cessation of symptoms" (de Graeff and Dean 2007).

pansexual An attraction to other people regardless of assigned sex at birth or gender identity.

Patient and Family Outcomes-Focused Inquiry for Developing Goals for Care A model for eliciting goals of care from patients and families based on the National Hospice and Palliative Care Organization's recommended outcomes for hospice and palliative care (Institute of Medicine and National Research Council 2003).

Patient and Family Outcomes-Focused Inquiry for Interdisciplinary Teams A model for structuring interdisciplinary/interprofessional team meetings around a list of questions designed to keep the team focused on outcomes of care; based on the National Hospice and Palliative Care Organization's recommended outcomes for hospice and palliative care (Institute of Medicine and National Research Council 2003).

patient-care skills The skills needed by a patient and/or caregiver to support the patient in meeting bathing, dressing, feeding, transferring, toileting, and transportation needs.

patient centered An approach in which the patient rather than the health care provider directs the goals and focus of care.

perceptual barriers to care Fears, misperceptions, and concerns about palliative care and hospice care, either in general or specifically as they relate to one's status as an LGBTQ individual.

physical examination "A physical examination usually includes: Inspection (looking at the body), Palpation (feeling the body with fingers or hands), Auscultation (listening to sounds), and Percussion (producing sounds, usually by tapping on specific areas of the body)" (National Library of Medicine 2015c).

plan of care "A [clinician's] written plan describing the type and frequency of services and care a particular patient needs" (Medicare Interactive 2016b). A plan "based on the identified and expressed preferences, values, goals, and needs of the patient and family and . . . developed with professional guidance and support for patient/family decision making" (National Consensus Project for Quality Palliative Care 2013).

power imbalance "An unequal relationship, such as between a [health care provider] and [patient], due to more power or prestige from one party, making the other party less free or more dependent in regard to initially making independent choices" (Gladding 2011). (Note: I have replaced Gladding's terms *counselor* and *client* with the terms *health care provider* and *patient*.)

presence "(1) A mode of being available in a situation with the wholeness of one's individual being; a gift of self that can be given freely, invoked, or evoked. (2) [A] nursing intervention from the Nursing Interventions Classification (NIC) defined as being with another, both physically and psychologically, during times of need" (*Mosby's Medical Dictionary* 2009).

prognosis "A forecast of the probable course and/or outcome of a disease" (*Stedman's Medical Dictionary* 2006).

psychological distress "A range of symptoms and experiences of a person's internal life that are commonly held to be troubling, confusing, or out of the ordinary" (American Psychiatric Association 2013b).

psychosocial assessment "An evaluation of a person's mental health, social status, and functional capacity within the community, generally conducted by . . . social workers" (*Mosby's Medical Dictionary* 2009).

psychosocial history A patient history "involving both psychological and social aspects; age, education, [relational] and related aspects of a person's history" (*Stedman's Medical Dictionary* 2006). (Note: I have replaced the term *marital* with the more inclusive term *relational*.)

quality of life "A patient's general well-being, including mental status, stress level, sexual function, and self-perceived health status" (*Stedman's Medical Dictionary* 2006).

rapport "A conscious feeling of harmonious accord, trust, empathy, and mutual responsiveness between two or more people (health care provider and patient) that fosters the therapeutic process" (*Stedman's Medical Dictionary* 2006).

reflection A technique in which the health care provider rephrases or verbalizes what the patient appears to be feeling in an effort to convey empathy (Gladding 2011).

right to self-determination Under the 1990 Patient Self-Determination Act, the federal government formally recognized that individuals have a right "to decide now about the types and extent of medical care they want to accept or refuse if they become unable to make those decisions due to illness" (American Cancer Society 2015).

scope of practice "What a health professional can and cannot do to or for a patient is dependent on that health professional's scope of practice (SOP), which is defined by state boards of medicine, boards of nursing, etc., oftentimes with the guidance or instruction (via statute) of the state's legislature. State legislatures consistently consider [a] health care professional's ability to prescribe, dispense and/or administer drugs, to sign evaluations and/or certifications (such as death certificates), to allow admitting or clinical privileges at a health care facility, how a health professional can be addressed and what information they must wear on their badge, how they are reimbursed, whether they can independently run a health clinic, how they can maintain licensure, where they can practice, which board they fall under and whether to create or dismember other medical boards, the ability of the health professional to advertise and what that advertisement can or cannot look like, etc." (National Conference of State Legislatures 2013).

self-awareness "An ongoing process in life of recognizing thoughts, emotions, senses, and behaviors that influence a person on multiple levels" (Gladding 2011).

self-disclosure "A conscious, intentional technique in which clinicians share information about their lives outside the counseling relationship" (Gladding 2011).

sex "The biological and physiological characteristics that define men and women" (WHO 2016a).

sexual behavior Acts engaged in by an individual toward the goal of sexual pleasure, reproduction, or both.

sexual expression The way in which individuals express their sexual desires alone and with partners. It is more than "sex": "Sexual expression is a form of communication through which we give and receive pleasure and emotion. It has a wide range of possibilities—from sharing fun activities, feelings and thoughts, warm touch or hugs, to physical intimacy. It is expressed both individually and in relationships throughout life" (McKinley Health Center 2009).

sexual health "A state of physical, emotional, mental and social well-being in relation to sexuality; it is not merely the absence of disease, dysfunction or infirmity. Sexual health requires a positive and respectful approach to sexuality and sexual relationships, as well as the possibility of having pleasurable and safe sexual experiences, free of coercion, discrimination and violence. For sexual health to be attained and maintained, the sexual rights of all persons must be respected, protected and fulfilled" (WHO 2006, 2010).

sexuality "A central aspect of being human throughout life encompasses sex, gender identities and roles, sexual orientation, eroticism, pleasure, intimacy and reproduction. Sexuality is experienced and expressed in thoughts, fantasies, desires, beliefs, attitudes, values, behaviors, practices, roles and relationships. While sexuality can include all of these dimensions, not all of them are always experienced or expressed. Sexuality is influenced by the interaction of biological, psychological, social, economic, political, cultural, legal, historical, religious and spiritual factors" (WHO 2006, 2010).

sexual orientation A person's sexual and emotional attraction toward men, women, or both.

shared decision making "A collaborative process that allows patients and their providers to make health care decisions together, taking into account the best scientific evidence available, as well as the patient's values and preferences. [Shared decision making] honors both the provider's expert knowledge and the patient's right to be fully informed of all care options and the potential harms and benefits. This process provides patients with the support they need to make the best individualized care decisions, while allowing providers to feel confident in the care they prescribe" (Informed Medical Decisions Foundation n.d.).

signs and symptoms of imminent death Changes seen in a patient's eating and drinking as well as in their neurological, integumentary (skin), respiratory, excretory, cardiac, and circulatory systems indicative of approaching death.

silence A purposeful absence of speaking on the part of the health care provider that is designed to encourage the patient to feel, reflect, and, if they choose to do so, speak.

sodomy laws Laws that make anal and/or oral sex between two adults illegal.

spiritual/existential assessment "Refers to a more extensive process of active listening to a patient's story conducted by a board-certified chaplain that summarizes the needs and resources that emerge in that process. The chaplain's summary should include a spiritual care plan with expected outcomes that is then communicated to the rest of the treatment team" (Puchalski et al. 2009).

spiritual/existential distress "(1) Discomfort related to religious, intellectual, or cultural concerns; (2) a nursing diagnosis approved by the North American Nursing Diagnosis Association, defined as disruption in the life principle that pervades a person's entire being and that integrates and transcends his or her biological and psychosocial nature. The person experiencing spiritual distress may express concern with the meaning of life and death, question the meaning of suffering or of his or her own existence, verbalize inner conflict about beliefs, express anger toward God or other Supreme Being (however defined), or actively seek spiritual assistance" (*Miller-Keane Encyclopedia and Dictionary of Medicine* 2003).

spiritual/existential history "Spiritual history-taking is the process of interviewing a patient in order to come to a better understanding of [his or her] spiritual needs and resources. A spiritual history can be integrated into existing formats such as the social history section of the clinical database. . . . The information from the history permits the clinician to understand how spiritual concerns could either complement or complicate the patient's overall care" (Puchalski et al. 2009).

suicidal ideation (also *suicidal ideas*) "Thoughts about self-harm, with deliberate consideration or planning of possible techniques of causing one's own death" (American Psychiatric Association 2013b).

symptom "A subjective manifestation of a pathological condition. Symptoms are reported by the affected individual rather than observed by the examiner" (American Psychiatric Association 2013b).

symptom management "An approach to palliative care that treats the symptoms rather than the cause of a condition. Its focus includes confusion, dizziness, fatigue, incontinence, nausea, shortness of breath, vomiting, and weakness" (*Medical Dictionary* 2009).

touch The use of physical contact by a health care provider to convey support to a patient. Touch should be used only with the express consent of the patient and should be offered in an effort to meet the patient's needs, not the needs of the health care provider.

transgender A person who is part of "the broad spectrum of individuals who transiently or permanently identify with a gender different from" the sex they were assigned at birth (American Psychiatric Association 2013b). Often abbreviated as "trans."

unconscious bias An attitude or preference that a health care provider feels toward or against an individual or group of people without consciously choosing to feel that way.

weakness "Weakness may be all over the body or in only one area. Weakness is more noticeable when it is in one area. [When] you . . . feel weak but have no real loss of strength, [t]his is called subjective weakness. . . . Or, you may have a loss of strength that can be noted on a physical exam. This is called objective weakness" (National Library of Medicine 2014).

weight loss "Unexplained weight loss is a decrease in body weight, when you did not try to lose the weight on your own. . . . Unintentional weight loss is loss of 10 pounds OR 5 percent of your normal body weight over 6 to 12 months or less without knowing the reason" (National Library of Medicine 2015d).

will "A will (last will and testament) [is a] . . . financial document [that] allow[s] [patients] to plan who receives [their] financial assets and property" (National Hospice and Palliative Care Organization 2016).

REFERENCES

Adelson, S., and W. Bockting. 2014. *Caring for Gender Dysphoric Children and Adolescents.* Document for National LGBT Health Education Center webinar. Boston: Fenway Institute. Accessed January 7, 2016. http://www.lgbthealtheducation.org/wp-content/uploads/Caring-for-Gender-Dysphoric-Children-and-Adolescents.pdf.

Administration for Community Living. n.d. *Advance Care Planning for Serious Illness.* Accessed March 9, 2016. http://www.eldercare.gov/Eldercare.NET/Public/Resources/Advanced_Care/docs/AdvancedCarePlanning.pdf.

Akinola, O., J. Baru, and S. Marks. 2015. *Fast Facts and Concepts #297: Terminal Hemorrhage Preparation and Management.* Accessed May 28, 2016. http://www.mypcnow.org/#!blank/zye98.

Almack, K., A. Yip, J. Seymour, A. Sargeant, A. Patterson, and M. Makita. 2014. *The Last Outing: Exploring End of Life Experiences and Care Needs in the Lives of Older LGBT People.* Accessed April 1, 2016. http://www.nottingham.ac.uk/research/groups/srcc/documents/projects/srcc project-report-last-outing.pdf.

Altilio, T., and S. Otis-Green, eds. 2011. *Oxford Textbook of Palliative Social Work.* New York: Oxford University Press.

Altilio, T., S. Otis-Green, and C. Dahlin. 2008. "Applying the National Quality Forum Preferred Practices for Palliative and Hospice Care: A Social Work Perspective." *Journal of Social Work in End-of-Life and Palliative Care* 4 (1): 3–16.

American Academy of Family Physicians (AAFP). n.d. *Recommended Curriculum Guidelines for Family Medicine Residents: Lesbian, Gay, Bisexual, Transgender Health.* Accessed November 4, 2015. http://www.aafp.org/dam/AAFP/documents/medical_education_residency/program_directors/Reprint289D_LGBT.pdf.

American Academy of Hospice and Palliative Medicine (AAHPM). 2009. *Hospice and Palliative Medicine Core Competencies, Version 2.3.* Accessed October 30, 2015. http://aahpm.org/uploads/education/competencies/Competencies%20v.%202.3.pdf.

———. 2014. "Palliative Sedation Position Statement." Accessed February 3, 2016. http://aahpm.org/positions/palliative-sedation.

———. n.d. "Certification for Hospice and Palliative Medicine Specialists." Accessed January 4, 2016. http://aahpm.org/education/certification.

American Cancer Society. 2015. "The Patient Self-Determination Act." Accessed January 28, 2016. http://www.cancer.org/treatment/findingandpayingfortreatment/understandingfinancialandlegalmatters/advancedirectives/advance-directives-patient-self-determination-act.

American Civil Liberties Union (ACLU). n.d. *Getting Rid of Sodomy Laws: History and Strategy That Led to the Lawrence Decision.* Accessed January 12, 2016. https://www.aclu.org/getting-rid-sodomy-laws-history-and-strategy-led-lawrence-decision.

American Medical Association (AMA). 2001. *Code of Medical Ethics of the American Medical Association.* Accessed April 13, 2016. http://www .ama-assn.org/ama/pub/physician-resources/medical-ethics/code -medical-ethics.page.

American Nurses Association (ANA). 2015. *Code of Ethics for Nurses with Interpretive Statements.* Accessed April 1, 2016. http://www.nursing world.org/MainMenuCategories/EthicsStandards/CodeofEthics forNurses/Code-of-Ethics-For-Nurses.html.

American Pain Society. 2008. *Principles of Analgesic Use in the Treatment of Acute Pain and Cancer Pain.* 6th ed. Glenview, Ill.: American Pain Society.

———. 2016. "Clinical Practice Guidelines." Accessed May 27, 2016. http://americanpainsociety.org/education/guidelines/overview.

American Psychiatric Association (APA). 2013a. "Gender Dysphoria." Accessed May 2, 2016. http://www.dsm5.org/documents/gender%20 dysphoria%20fact%20sheet.pdf.

———. 2013b. "Glossary of Technical Terms." In *Diagnostic and Statistical Manual of Mental Disorders,* ed. American Psychiatric Association. 5th ed. Arlington, Va.: American Psychiatric Publishing.

American Psychological Association. 2008. *Answers to Your Questions: For a Better Understanding of Sexual Orientation and Homosexuality.* Accessed June 25, 2016. http://www.apa.org/topics/lgbt/orientation.pdf.

Association of American Medical Colleges (AAMC). 2014. Implementing Curricular and Institutional Climate Changes to Improve Health Care for Individuals Who Are LGBT, Gender Nonconforming, or Born with DSD: A Resource for Medical Educators. Accessed May 28, 2016. https://lgbt.ucsf.edu/sites/lgbt.ucsf.edu/files/wysiwyg/AAMC_LGBT -DSD%20Report%202014.pdf.

Association of Professional Chaplains. 2000. *Associate of Professional Chaplains Code of Ethics.* Accessed April 12, 2016. http://www.profes sionalchaplains.org/files/professional_standards/professional_ethics/ apc_code_of_ethics.pdf.

Austin Community College. "Nursing Process: Planning Outcome Oriented Care." Accessed February 18, 2016. http://www.austincc.edu/adnlev1/ rnsg1413online/mod_nursing_process/outcome.html.

Barry, M., and S. Edgman-Levitan. 2012. "Shared Decision-Making: The Pinnacle of Patient-Centered Care." *New England Journal of Medicine* 366: 780–781. doi: 10.1056/NEJMp1109283.

Beauchamp, T., and J. Childress. 2013. *Principles of Biomedical Ethics.* 7th ed. New York: Oxford University Press.

Benbassat, J., and R. Baumal. 2005. "Enhancing Self-Awareness in Medical Students: An Overview of Teaching Approaches." *Academic Medicine* 80 (2): 156–161. doi: 10.1097/00001888-200502000-00010.

Board of Chaplaincy Certification. n.d. "Competencies of the Certified Hospice and Palliative Care Chaplain." Accessed January 4, 2016. http://bcci.professionalchaplains.org/content.asp?pl=45&sl=42& contentid=49.

Bristowe, K., S. Marshall, and R. Harding. 2016. "The Bereavement Experiences of Lesbian, Gay, Bisexual and/or Trans People Who Have Lost a Partner: A Systematic Review, Thematic Synthesis and Modelling of the Literature." *Palliative Medicine.* March 4. doi: 10.1177/026921631 6634601.

Bruera, E., N. Kuehn, M. J. Miller, P. Selmser, and K. Macmillan. 1991. "The Edmonton Symptom Assessment System (ESAS): A Simple Method for the Assessment of Palliative Care Patients." *Journal of Palliative Care* 7 (2): 6–9.

Byock, I. R. 1994. "A Working Set of Landmarks and Developmental Taskwork." Accessed March 29, 2016. http://www.mywhatever.com/cif writer/content/18/dw53.html.

Byock, I. R., and M. P. Merriman. 1998. "Measuring Quality of Life for Patients with Terminal Illness: The Missoula-VITAS Quality of Life Index." *Palliative Medicine* 12: 231–244.

———. n.d. "The Missoula-VITAS Quality of Life Index (MVQOLI) ©: An Outcome Measure for Palliative Care: Guide to Using the MVQOLI." Accessed March 29, 2016. http://www.npcrc.org/files/ news/missoula_vitas_quality_of_life_index.pdf.

California State University Institute for Palliative Care and the Healthcare Chaplaincy Network. 2015. "Palliative Care Competency Framework for Chaplains." Accessed January 25, 2016. https://csupalliativecare.org/ programs/chap-competencies/.

Cambridge Dictionary Online. n.d. S.v. "assumption." Accessed January 28, 2016. http://dictionary.cambridge.org/us/dictionary/english/ assumption.

Candrian, C., and H. Lum. 2015. "Lesbian, Gay, Bisexual, and Transgender Communication." In *Textbook of Palliative Care Communication,* ed. E. Wittenberg, B. Ferrell, J. Goldsmith, T. Smith, M. Glajchen, and G. Handzo. New York: Oxford University Press.

Centers for Disease Control [CDC]. 2015. "Tips from Former Smokers: Lesbian, Gay, Bisexual, and Transgender (LGBT)." Accessed May 5, 2016. http://www.cdc.gov/tobacco/campaign/tips/groups/lgbt.html.

———. 2016. "HIV among Transgender People." Accessed May 28, 2016. http://www.cdc.gov/hiv/group/gender/transgender/.

Centers for Medicaid and Medicare Services (CMS). 2015a. "Local Coverage Determination: Hospice Determining TERMINAL Status - L34538." Accessed March 1, 2016. https://www.cms.gov/medicare-coverage -database/details/lcd-details.x? LCDId=34538&ContrId=236&ver= 3&ContrVer=2&CntrctrSelected=236*2&Cntrctr=236&name=CGS+ Administrators%2c+LLC+(15004%2c+HHH+MAC)&DocType= Active&LCntrctr=236*2&bc=AgACAAQAAAAAAA%3d%3d&.

———. 2015b. *State Operations Manual: Appendix M—Guidance to Surveyors: Hospice.* Accessed February 17, 2016. https://www.cms.gov/Regula tions-and-Guidance/Guidance/Manuals/Downloads/som107ap_m_ hospice.pdf.

Center to Advance Palliative Care. 2010. "Palliative Sedation: Myth vs. Fact." Accessed May 25, 2016. https://www.capc.org/about/press-media/press-releases/2010-1-6/palliative-sedation-myth-vs-fact/.

———. 2012a. "Get Palliative Care: Glossary." Accessed January 27, 2016. https://getpalliativecare.org/whatis/glossary/.

———. 2012b. "Get Palliative Care: Handouts for Patients and Families." Accessed January 28, 2016. https://getpalliativecare.org/handouts-for-patients-and-families/.

Chai, E., D. Meier, J. Morris, and S. Goldhirsch, eds. 2014. *Geriatric Palliative Care*. New York: Oxford University Press.

Charles, C., A. Gafni, and T. Whelan. 1999. "Decision-Making in the Physician-Patient Encounter: Revisiting the Shared Treatment Decision-Making Model." *Social Science & Medicine* 49 (5): 651–661. Accessed July 8, 2016. http://dx.doi.org/10.1016/S0277-9536(99)00145-8.

Cherny, N., M. Fallon, S. Kaasa, R. Portenoy, and D. Currow, eds. 2015. *Oxford Textbook of Palliative Medicine*. 5th ed. New York: Oxford University Press.

City of Orlando. 2016. "Victims' Names." Accessed June 20, 2016. http://www.cityoforlando.net/blog/victims/.

Coble, C. 2015. "Do Sodomy Laws Still Exist?" *FindLaw Blotter*. Accessed January 13, 2016. http://blogs.findlaw.com/blotter/2015/09/do-sodomy-laws-still-exist.html.

Dahlin, C., P. Coyne, and B. Ferrell, eds. 2016. *Advanced Practice Palliative Nursing*. New York: Oxford University Press.

Dahlin, C., and M. Lynch. 2003. *HPNA Position Statement: Palliative Sedation at End of Life*. Hospice and Palliative Nurses Association. Accessed May 26, 2016. https://www.hpna.org/filemaintenance_view.aspx?ID=26.

De Bord, J., W. Burke, and D. Dudzinski. 2013. "Ethics in Medicine: Confidentiality." Accessed January 27, 2016. https://depts.washington.edu/bioethx/topics/confiden.html.

de Graeff, A., and M. Dean. 2007. "Palliative Sedation Therapy in the Last Weeks of Life: A Literature Review and Recommendations for Standards." *Journal of Palliative Medicine* 10: 67–85.

DeMeester, R., F. Lopez, J. Moore, M. Cook, and M. Chin. 2016. "A Model of Organizational Context and Shared Decision-Making: Application to LGBT Racial and Ethnic Minority Patients." *Journal of General Internal Medicine* 31 (6): 651–662.

Eisenhower, D. 1953. "Television Report to the American People by the President and Members of the Cabinet." June 3, 1953. Online at Gerhard Peters and John T. Woolley, The American Presidency Project. Accessed March 15, 2016. http://www.presidency.ucsb.edu/ws/?pid=9868.

Elwyn, G., C. Dehlendorf, R. M. Epstein, K. Marrin, J. White, D. L. Frosch, et al. 2014. "Shared Decision-Making and Motivational Interviewing: Achieving Patient-Centered Care across the Spectrum of Health care Problems." *Annals of Family Medicine* 12 (3): 270–275.

Elwyn, G., D. Frosch, R. Thomson, N. Joseph-Williams, A. Lloyd, P. Kinnersley, E. Cording, et al. 2012. "Shared Decision-Making: A Model

for Clinical Practice." *Journal of General Internal Medicine* 27 (10):
1361–1367. http://doi.org/10.1007/s11606-012-2077-6.

Emanuel, L., C. von Gunten, F. Ferris, and J. Hauser, eds. 1999–2011.
The Education in Palliative and End-of-Life Care (EPEC) Curriculum.
© The EPEC Program, 1999–2011. http://www.epec.net.

Erickson-Schroth, Laura. 2014. *Trans Bodies, Trans Selves: A Resource for
the Transgender Community.* New York: Oxford University Press.

Fenway Institute and the Center for American Progress. 2014. *Asking
Patients Questions about Sexual Orientation and Gender Identity in
Clinical Settings: A Study in Four Health Centers.* Accessed May 28,
2016. http://thefenwayinstitute.org/wp-content/uploads/COM228_
SOGI_CHARN_WhitePaper.pdf.

Ferrell, B., ed. 2015. *Pediatric Palliative Care.* New York: Oxford University
Press.

Ferrell, B., N. Coyle, and J. Paice, eds. 2015a. *Oxford Textbook of Palliative
Nursing.* 4th ed. New York: Oxford University Press.

———. 2015b. *Social Aspects of Palliative Care.* New York: Oxford University
Press.

Ferrer, R., and J. Gill. 2013. "Shared Decision-Making, Contextualized."
Annals of Family Medicine 11: 303–305.

Gale Encyclopedia of Medicine. 2008. S.v. "pain management." Accessed
January 28, 2016. http://medical-dictionary.thefreedictionary.com/
pain+management.

Gawande, Atul. 2014. *Being Mortal: Medicine and What Matters in the End.*
New York: Metropolitan Books/Henry Holt and Company.

Gendered Innovations. n.d. "Gender." Accessed April 28, 2016. https://
genderedinnovations.stanford.edu/terms/gender.html.

Gender Equity Resource Center. 2013. "Definition of Terms." Accessed
January 26, 2016. http://ejce.berkeley.edu/geneq/resources/lgbtq
-resources/definition-terms.

GenoPro. 2016a. "Introduction to the Genogram." Accessed February 8,
2016. http://www.genopro.com/genogram/.

———. 2016b. "Rules to Build Genograms." Accessed February 8, 2016.
http://www.genopro.com/genogram/rules/.

Gibson, S. 2016. "The Advanced Practice Registered Nurse in Hospice."
In *Advanced Practice Palliative Nursing,* ed. C. Dahlin, P. Coyne, and B.
Ferrell. New York: Oxford University Press.

Gladding, S. 2011. *The Counseling Dictionary: Concise Definitions of Frequently
Used Terms.* 3rd ed. Upper Saddle River, N.J.: Pearson Education.

Gleason, K. M., H. Brake, V. Agramonte, and C. Perfetti. 2012. *Medications at
Transitions and Clinical Handoffs (MATCH) Toolkit for Medication Reconciliation.* Rev. ed. Prepared by the Island Peer Review Organization, under
Contract No. HHSA290200900013C. AHRQ Publication No. 11(12)-
0059. Rockville, Md.: Agency for Healthcare Research and Quality.

Golley, L. 2012. *Cultural Issues around End of Life.* University of Washington Medical Center, Interpreter Services. Accessed February 9, 2016.
http://www.uwmedicine.org/uw-medical-center/documents/Cultural
-Issues-around-End-of-Life.pdf.

Grant, J., L. Mottet, J. Tanis, J. Harrison, J. Herman, and M. Keisling. 2011. *Injustice at Every Turn: A Report of the National Transgender Discrimination Survey*. Washington, D.C.: National Center for Transgender Equality and National Gay and Lesbian Task Force. Accessed January 12, 2016. http://www.thetaskforce.org/static_html/downloads/reports/reports/ntds_full.pdf.

Griebling, T. 2016. "Sexuality and Aging: A Focus on Lesbian, Gay, Bisexual, and Transgender (LGBT) Needs in Palliative and End of Life Care." *Current Opinion in Supportive & Palliative Care* 10 (1): 95–101.

Harding, R., E. Epiphaniou, and J. Chidgey-Clark. 2012. "Needs, Experiences, and Preferences of Sexual Minorities for End-of-Life Care and Palliative Care: A Systematic Review." *Journal of Palliative Medicine* 15 (5): 602–611.

Hay, A., and S. Johnson. 2001. *Fundamental Skills and Knowledge for Hospice and Palliative Care Social Workers: Competency-Based Education for Social Workers*. Arlington, Va.: National Hospice and Palliative Care Organization.

Hilliard, R. 2012. "Psychosocial Documentation: A Plan to Support ADRs." *NHPCO Newsline*, June. Accessed March 17, 2016. http://www.nhpco.org/sites/default/files/public/newsline/2012/NL_June2012.pdf.

Hospice and Palliative Credentialing Center (HPCC). 2016a. "Advanced Certified Hospice and Palliative Nurse." Accessed January 4, 2016. http://hpcc.advancingexpertcare.org/competence/aprn-achpn/.

———. 2016b. "Certified Hospice and Palliative Nurse." Accessed January 4, 2016. http://hpcc.advancingexpertcare.org/competence/rn-chpn/.

Hospice Medical Director Certification Board. 2013. "Eligibility Requirements." Accessed May 17, 2016. http://www.hmdcb.org/about-the-exam/default/eligibility.html.

Hughes, M., and C. Cartwright. 2015. "Lesbian, Gay, Bisexual and Transgender People's Attitudes to End-of-Life Decision-Making and Advance Care Planning." *Australasian Journal on Ageing* 34 (S2): 39–43.

Human Rights Campaign. n.d. "Hate Crimes Timeline." Accessed January 12, 2016. http://www.hrc.org/resources/hate-crimes-timeline.

Human Rights Campaign Foundation. 2016. *Corporate Equality Index 2016: Criteria Updates and Toolkit for Success*. Accessed April 13, 2016. http://hrc-assets.s3-website-us-east-1.amazonaws.com//files/assets/resources/CEIToolkit-2016-REV2.pdf.

Informed Medical Decisions Foundation. n.d. "Why Shared Decision-Making?" Accessed February 1, 2016. http://www.informedmedicaldecisions.org/what-is-shared-decision-making/.

Institute for Healthcare Improvement. 2016. "Medication Reconciliation to Prevent Adverse Drug Events." Accessed May 28, 2016. http://www.ihi.org/topics/adesmedicationreconciliation/Pages/default.aspx.

Institute of Medicine (IOM). 1993. *Access to Health Care in America*. Washington, D.C.: National Academies Press.

———. 2011. *The Health of Lesbian, Gay, Bisexual, and Transgender (LGBT) People: Building a Foundation for Better Understanding*. Washington, D.C.: National Academies Press. Accessed May 28, 2016. http://www

.nap.edu/login.php?record_id=13128&page=http%3A%2F%2Fwww
.nap.edu%2Fdownload%2F13128.

———. 2013. *Delivering High-Quality Cancer Care: Charting a New Course for a System in Crisis*. Washington, D.C.: National Academies Press.

———. 2015. *Dying in America: Improving Quality and Honoring Individual Preferences Near the End of Life*. Washington, D.C.: National Academies Press.

Institute of Medicine and National Research Council. 2003. *Describing Death in America: What We Need to Know*. Washington, D.C.: National Academies Press. doi:10.17226/10619.

International Association for the Study of Pain. 2012. "IASP Taxonomy." Accessed May 28, 2016. http://www.iasp-pain.org/Taxonomy#Pain.

Intersex Society of North America. 2008. "What Is Intersex?" Accessed on May 25, 2016. http://www.isna.org/faq/what_is_intersex.

Joint Commission. 2011. *Advancing Effective Communication, Cultural Competence, and Patient- and Family-Centered Care for the Lesbian, Gay, Bisexual, and Transgender (LGBT) Community: A Field Guide*. Oakbrook Terrace, Ill.: Joint Commission. Accessed November 4, 2015. http://www.jointcommission.org/assets/1/18/LGBTFieldGuide_WEB_LINKED_VER.pdf.

Kaleem, J. 2016. "Orthodox Rabbi Addresses Transgender Issues." Accessed March 17, 2016. http://www.jewishjournal.com/religion/article/orthodox_rabbi_addresses_transgender_issues.

Kerr, M. 2000. "One Family's Story: A Primer on Bowen Theory." Bowen Center for the Study of the Family. Accessed February 5, 2016. http://www.thebowencenter.org.

Knight, S. n.d. *EndLink: An Internet-Based End of Life Care Education Program. Part I: How to Assess Spirituality*. Accessed April 11, 2016. http://endlink.lurie.northwestern.edu/religion_spirituality/part_one.pdf.

Knight, S., and C. von Gunten. 2004. *Module 3: Whole-Patient Assessment: Nine Dimensions*. EndLink: Resource for End of Life Care Education. Accessed January 22, 2016. http://www.endoflife.northwestern.edu/whole_patient_assessment/step1.cfm.

Kroenke, K., R. Spitzer, and J. Williams. 2001. "The PHQ-9: Validity of a Brief Depression Severity Measure." *Journal of General Internal Medicine* 16: 606–613.

Lambda Legal. 2010. *When Health Care Isn't Caring: Lambda Legal's Survey of Discrimination against LGBT People and People with HIV*. New York: Lambda Legal. Accessed January 14, 2016. http://www.lambdalegal.org/health-care-report.

———. 2014. *Tools for Protecting Your Wishes for Your Funeral*. Accessed March 14, 2016. http://www.lambdalegal.org/sites/default/files/final_pp_ttp-2014-07_protecting-your-wishes-for-your-funeral.pdf.

LaRocca-Pitts, M. 2007. *A Spiritual History Tool*. Accessed January 28, 2016. http://www.professionalchaplains.org/files/resources/reading_room/spiritual_history_tool_fact_larocca_pitts.pdf.

Lau, D. T., J. D. Kasper, J. M. Hauser, C. Berdes, C. H. Chang, R. L. Berman, J. Masin-Peters, J. Paice, and L. Emanuel. 2009. "Family Caregiver Skills in Medication Management for Hospice Patients: A Qualitative Study to Define a Construct." *Journals of Gerontology Series B* 64: 799–807.

Lawton, A., J. White, and E. Fromme. 2014. "End-of-Life and Advance Care Planning Considerations for Lesbian, Gay, Bisexual, and Transgender Patients #275." *Journal of Palliative Medicine* 17 (1): 106–107.

Legal Information Institute. n.d. "Employment Discrimination: An Overview." Cornell University Law School. Accessed January 14, 2016. https://www.law.cornell.edu/wex/employment_discrimination.

Legare, F., D. Stacey, and IP Team. 2014. "IP-SDM Model." Accessed February 1, 2016. https://decisionaid.ohri.ca/docs/develop/IP-SDM -Model.pdf.

Limbo, R., and B. Davies. 2015. "Grief and Bereavement in Pediatric Palliative Care." In *Pediatric Palliative Care,* ed. B. Ferrell. New York: Oxford University Press.

Makoul, G., and M. L. Clayman. 2006. "An Integrative Model of Shared Decision-Making in Medical Encounters." *Patient Education and Counseling* 60 (3): 301–312. Accessed January 10, 2016. http://dx.doi .org/10.1016/j.pec.2005.06.010.

Maltoni, M., C. Pittureri, E. Scarpi, L. Piccinini, F. Martini, P. Turci, L. Montanari, O. Nanni, and D. Amadori. 2009. "Palliative Sedation Therapy Does Not Hasten Death: Results from a Prospective Multicenter Study." *Annals of Oncology* 20 (7): 1163–1169. Accessed February 2, 2016. doi: 10.1093/annonc/mdp048.

Massachusetts Executive Office of Public Safety. n.d. *A Firefighter's Guide to Educating Occupant(s) on the Hazards of Smoking and Home Oxygen Use.* Accessed February 25, 2016. http://www.mass.gov/eopss/docs/ dfs/osfm/pubed/flyers/ff-ed-guidelines.pdf.

Matzo, M. 2015. "Sexuality." In *Oxford Textbook of Palliative Nursing,* ed. B. Ferrell, N. Coyle, and J. Paice. 4th ed. New York: Oxford University Press.

Mayo Foundation for Medical Education and Research. n.d.a. "Symptoms: Shortness of Breath: Definition." Accessed January 27, 2016. http:// www.mayoclinic.org/symptoms/shortness-of-breath/basics/defini tion/sym-20050890.

———. n.d.b. "Stress Relief from Laughter? It's No Joke." *Healthy Lifestyle: Stress Management.* Accessed April 28, 2016. http://www.mayoclinic .org/healthy-lifestyle/stress-management/in-depth/stress-relief/ art-20044456.

Mazanec, P., and J. Panke. 2016. "Cultural Considerations in Palliative Care." In *Spiritual, Religious, and Cultural Aspects of Care,* ed. B. Ferrell. HPNA Palliative Nursing Manuals. New York: Oxford University Press.

McKinley Health Center. 2009. "Healthy Sexuality." University of Illinois at Urbana-Champaign. Accessed May 17, 2016. http://www.mckinley .illinois.edu/handouts/healthy_sexuality.htm.

Medical Dictionary. 2009. S.v. "open posture," "symptom management." Accessed January 28, 2016. http://medical-dictionary.thefree dictionary.com.

Medicare Interactive. 2016a. "Glossary." Accessed January 27, 2016. http://www.medicareinteractive.org/glossary.

———. 2016b. "Types of Medical Equipment Medicare Covers If You Live at Home." Accessed January 27, 2016. http://www.medicareinteractive .org/get-answers/medicare-covered-services/durable-medical-equipment -part-b/types-of-medical-equipment-medicare-covers-if-you-live-at-home.

MedicineNet. 2012. "Definition of Informed Consent." Accessed January 27, 2016. http://www.medicinenet.com/script/main/art.asp?articlekey=22414.

Merriam-Webster Dictionary. 2015. S.v. "belief." Accessed January 28, 2016. http://www.merriam-webster.com/dictionary/belief.

Miller-Keane Encyclopedia and Dictionary of Medicine, Nursing, and Allied Health. 2003. 7th ed. S.v. "distress." Accessed April 1, 2016. http:// medical-dictionary.thefreedictionary.com/distress.

Mosby's Medical Dictionary. 2009. 9th ed. S.v. "distress," "end-stage disease," "presence," "psychosocial assessment." Accessed April 1, 2016. http://medical-dictionary.thefreedictionary.com.

Movement Advancement Project. 2016. *Non-Discrimination Laws.* Accessed January 12, 2016. http://www.lgbtmap.org/equality-maps/ non_discrimination_laws.

Naierman, N., and J. Turner. 2012. "Debunking the Myths of Hospice." Accessed January 14, 2016. https://americanhospice.org/learning -about-hospice/debunking-the-myths-of-hospice/.

National Association of Social Workers (NASW). 2004. *NASW Standards for Social Work Practice in Palliative and End of Life Care.* Accessed January 4, 2016. http://www.naswdc.org/practice/standards/Palliative.asp.

———. 2007. *Indicators for the Achievement of the NASW Standards for Cultural Competence in Social Work Practice.* Accessed November 4, 2015. http://www.socialworkers.org/practice/standards/NASWCulturalStan dardsIndicators2006.pdf.

———. 2008. *Code of Ethics of the National Association of Social Workers.* Accessed April 12, 2016. https://www.socialworkers.org/pubs/code/ code.asp.

National Comprehensive Cancer Network. 2016. *NCCN Guidelines.* Accessed May 27, 2016. https://www.nccn.org/professionals/physician_ gls/f_guidelines.asp.

National Conference of State Legislatures. 2013. *Scope of Practice Overview.* Accessed January 28, 2016. http://www.ncsl.org/research/health/ scope-of-practice-overview.aspx.

National Consensus Project for Quality Palliative Care. 2013. *Clinical Practice Guidelines for Quality Palliative Care.* 3rd ed. Edited by C. Dahlin. Accessed May 25, 2016. http://www.nationalconsensusproject .org/Guidelines_Download2.aspx.

National Hospice and Palliative Care Organization (NHPCO). 2000. *Patient and Family Centered Care (PFC).* Accessed February 9, 2016.

http://www.nhpco.org/sites/default/files/public/quality/Standards/
PFC.pdf.

———. 2015a. "Hospice Care." Accessed January 28, 2016. http://www
.nhpco.org/about/hospice-care.

———. 2015b. "Sec. 418.106, Condition of Participation: Drugs and Bio-
logicals, Medical Supplies, and Durable Medical Equipment." In
*Medicare Hospice Conditions of Participation (CoPs): Compliance Guide
for Hospice Providers.*" Accessed March 8, 2016. http://www.nhpco
.org/sites/default/files/public/regulatory/Drug_disposal-COPS_by_
topic.pdf.

———. 2016. *End-of-Life Decisions.* Accessed February 25, 2016. http://
www.caringinfo.org/files/public/brochures/End-of-Life_Decisions.pdf.

———. n.d. *Medicare Hospice Conditions of Participation: Spiritual Caregiver.*
Accessed April 11, 2016. http://www.nhpco.org/sites/default/files/
public/regulatory/Spiritual_tip_sheet.pdf.

National LGBT Health Education Center. 2015. *Collecting Sexual Orientation and Gender Identity Data in Electronic Health Records: Taking the
Next Steps.* The Fenway Institute. Accessed May 27, 2016. http://
www.lgbthealtheducation.org/wp-content/uploads/Collecting-SOGI
-Data-in-EHRs-COM2111.pdf.

National Library of Medicine. 2014. "Weakness." In *MedlinePlus Medical
Encyclopedia.* National Institutes of Health. Accessed January 27, 2016.
https://www.nlm.nih.gov/medlineplus/ency/article/003174.htm.

———. 2015a. "Fatigue." In *MedlinePlus Medical Encyclopedia.* National
Institutes of Health. Accessed January 27, 2016. https://www.nlm
.nih.gov/medlineplus/ency/article/003088.htm.

———. 2015b. "Nausea and Vomiting—Adults." In *MedlinePlus Medical
Encyclopedia.* National Institutes of Health. Accessed January 27,
2016. https://www.nlm.nih.gov/medlineplus/ency/article/003117.htm.

———. 2015c. "Physical Examination." In *MedlinePlus Medical Encyclopedia.* National Institutes of Health. Accessed January 27, 2016. https://
www.nlm.nih.gov/medlineplus/ency/article/002274.htm.

———. 2015d. "Weight Loss—Unintentional." In *MedlinePlus Medical
Encyclopedia.* National Institutes of Health. Accessed January 27, 2016.
https://www.nlm.nih.gov/medlineplus/ency/article/003107.htm.

———. 2016. "Do-Not-Resuscitate Order." In *MedlinePlus Medical Encyclopedia.* National Institutes of Health. Accessed January 27, 2016.
https://www.nlm.nih.gov/medlineplus/ency/patientinstructions/
000473.htm.

National Palliative Care Research Center. 2013a. *Guidelines for Using the
Edmonton Symptom Assessment Scale.* Accessed February 18, 2016.
http://www.npcrc.org/files/news/edmonton_symptom_assessment_
scale.pdf.

———. 2013b. *Memorial Symptom Assessment Scale.* Accessed February 18,
2016. http://www.npcrc.org/files/news/memorial_symptom_assess
ment_scale.pdf.

National POLST Paradigm. 2015. "POLST and Advance Directives." Accessed May 28, 2016. http://www.polst.org/advance-care-planning/polst-and-advance-directives/.

———. 2016. "What Is POLST?" Accessed May 5, 2016. http://www.polst.org/.

National Quality Forum. 2012. *National Voluntary Consensus Standards: Palliative and End-of-Life Care — A Consensus Report.* Accessed May 28, 2016. http://www.qualityforum.org/Publications/2012/04/Palliative_Care_and_End-of-Life_Care%E2%80%94A_Consensus_Report.aspx.

Neville, S., and M. Henrickson. 2009. "The Constitution of 'Lavender Families': A LGB Perspective." *Journal of Clinical Nursing* 18 (6): 849–856.

O'Connor, A., D. Stacey, and M. Jacobsen. 2015. "Ottowa Personal Decision Guide." Ottawa Hospital Research Institute. Accessed February 3, 2016. https://decisionaid.ohri.ca/docs/das/OPDG.pdf.

Palliative Care Network of Wisconsin. 2016. *Palliative Care Fast Facts and Concepts.* Accessed May 27, 2016. http://www.mypcnow.org/fast-facts.

Paul, R., and K. Adamson. 1993. "Critical Thinking and the Nature of Prejudice." In R. Paul, *Critical Thinking: What Every Person Needs to Survive in a Rapidly Changing World.* Santa Rosa, Calif.: Foundation for Critical Thinking.

Paxton, S. 2015. *Palliative Care: Myths vs. Reality in the New Era of Healthcare.* Accessed January 14, 2016. https://www.ohca.org/data/convention_2015_pdfs/W38.pdf.

PEACE Project. 2016. *PEACE Hospice and Palliative Care Quality Measures.* Accessed May 27, 2016. https://www.med.unc.edu/pcare/resources/PEACE-Quality-Measures.

Peek, M., F. Lopez, H. Williams, L. Xu, M. McNulty, M. Acree, and J. Schneider. 2016. "Development of a Conceptual Framework for Understanding Shared Decision-Making among African-American LGBT Patients and Their Clinicians." *Journal of General Internal Medicine* 31 (6): 677–687. Accessed July 12, 2016. doi: 10. 1007/s11606-016-3616-3.

Periyakoil, V. n.d. "Palliative Care Case Study: Palliative Sedation." Stanford School of Medicine. Accessed February 3, 2016. https://palliative.stanford.edu/palliative-sedation/case-study/.

Portenoy, R., H. Thaler, A. Kornblith, J. Lepore, H. Friedlander-Klar, E. Kiyasu, K. Sobel, et al. 1994. "The Memorial Symptom Assessment Scale: An Instrument for the Evaluation of Symptom Prevalence, Characteristics and Distress." *European Journal of Cancer* 30A (9): 1326–1336.

Puchalski, C. 1996. "FICA Spiritual History Tool." GW Institute for Spirituality and Health. Accessed January 26, 2016. https://smhs.gwu.edu/gwish/clinical/fica/spiritual-history-tool.

———. 2014. "The FICA Spiritual History Tool #274." *Journal of Palliative Medicine* 17 (1): 105–106.

Puchalski, C., B. Ferrell, R. Virani, S. Otis-Green, P. Baird, J. Bull, H. Chochinov, et al. 2009. "Improving the Quality of Spiritual Care as a Dimension of Palliative Care: The Report of the Consensus Conference."

Journal of Palliative Medicine 12 (10): 885–904. doi:10.1089/jpm
.2009.0142.

Rawlings, D. 2012. "End-of-Life Care Considerations for Gay, Lesbian,
Bisexual, and Transgender Individuals." *International Journal of Palliative Nursing* 18 (1): 29–34.

Redelman, M. 2008. "Is There a Place for Sexuality in the Holistic Care
of Patients in the Palliative Care Phase of Life?" *American Journal of
Hospice and Palliative Medicine* 25: 366–371.

Ross, D., and C. Alexander. 2001. "Management of Common Symptoms
in Terminally Ill Patients, Part II: Constipation, Delirium, and Dyspnea."
American Family Physician 64 (6): 1019–1026.

Sandilands, T. n.d. "Examples of a Mitigation Plan." Chron.com [*Houston
Chronicle*]. Accessed May 25, 2016. http://smallbusiness.chron.com/
examples-mitigation-plan-24507.html.

Schildmann, E., and J. Schildmann. 2014. "Palliative Sedation Therapy: A
Systematic Literature Review and Critical Appraisal of Available Guidance on Indication and Decision Making." *Journal of Palliative Medicine* 17
(5): 601–611. Accessed March 16, 2016. doi:10.1089/jpm.2013.0511.

Segen's Medical Dictionary. 2012. S.v. "sleep disturbance." Accessed January 28, 2016. http://medical-dictionary.thefreedictionary.com/
Sleep+disturbance.

Sieck, C., M. Johansen, and J. Stewart. 2016. "Inter-professional Shared
Decision-Making: Increasing the "Shared" in Shared Decision-Making." *International Journal of Healthcare* 2 (1). Accessed February 1,
2016. http://dx.doi.org/10.5430/ijh.v2n1p1.

Sinclair, C., J. Kalender-Rich, T. Griebling, and K. Porter-Williamson.
2015. "Palliative Care of Urologic Patients at End of Life." *Clinics in
Geriatric Medicine* 31: 667–678.

Smolinski, K., and Y. Colón. 2011. "Palliative Care with Lesbian, Gay, Bisexual, and Transgender Persons." In *Oxford Textbook of Palliative Social
Work,* ed. T. Altilio and S. Otis-Green. New York: Oxford University Press.

Stark, M., and J. J. Fins. 2013. "What's Not Being Shared in Shared Decision-Making?" *Hastings Center Report* 43 (4): 13–16.

Stedman's Medical Dictionary. 2006. 28th ed. Philadelphia: Wolters Kluwer
Health. Accessed January 26, 2016. http://www.medilexicon.com/
medicaldictionary.php.

Steinmetz, K. 2014. "This Is What 'Cisgender' Means." *Time,* December
23, 2014. Accessed January 14, 2016. http://time.com/3636430/
cisgender-definition/.

Sulmasy, D. 2006. "Spiritual Issues in the Care of Dying Patients: '. . . It's
Okay between Me and God.'" *Journal of the American Medical Association* 296 (1): 1385–1392.

Tan, J., L. Xu, F. Lopez, J. Jia, M. Pho, K. Kim, and M. Chin. 2016. "Shared
Decision-Making among Clinicians and Asian American and Pacific
Islander Sexual and Gender Minorities: An Intersectional Approach
to Address a Critical Care Gap." *LGBT Health* 3 (5): 327–334.
Accessed October 1, 2016. doi:10.1089/lgbt.2015.0143.

Tate, C., J. Ledbetter, and C. Youssef. 2013. "A Two-Question Method for Assessing Gender Categories in the Social and Medical Sciences." *Journal of Sex Research* 50 (8): 767–776. doi: 10.1080/00224499 .2012.690110.

Teich, Nicholas M. 2012. *Transgender 101: A Simple Guide to a Complex Issue.* New York: Columbia University Press.

Texas A&M AgriLife Extension. n.d. *Improving Independence in the Home Environment: Assessment and Intervention.* Reproduced from *Assessment and Intervention of the Home Environment for Older Persons,* Center for Therapeutic Applications of Technology, University of Buffalo. Accessed February 2, 2016. http://fcs.tamu.edu/files/2015/01/improving -independence-in-the-home-environment.pdf.

Torres, V. n.d. "Gay Events Timeline: 1970–1999." Sexual Orientation Issues in the News, USC Annenberg School for Communication. Accessed January 12, 2016. https://www.usc.edu/schools/annenberg/ asc/projects/soin/enhancingCurricula/timeline.html.

Trans Student Educational Resources. 2016. "Gender Pronouns." Designed by L. Pan. Accessed June 14, 2016. http://www.transstudent.org/ pronounsgraphic.jpg.

University of California, Davis. 2015. *LGBTQIA Resource Center Glossary.* Accessed on May 25, 2016. http://lgbtqia.ucdavis.edu/educated/ glossary.html.

U.S. Department of Health and Human Services. 2003. *HIPAA Privacy Rule at 45 CFR 164.510(b).* Accessed January 25, 2016. https://www .gpo.gov/fdsys/pkg/CFR-2003-title45-vol1/xml/CFR-2003-title45 -vol1-sec164-510.xml.

U.S. Department of Housing and Urban Development (HUD). 2011. *Department of Housing and Urban Development [Docket No. FR-5600-N-01] Notice of HUD's Fiscal Year (FY) 2012 Notice of Funding Availability (NOFA) Policy Requirements and General Section to HUD's FY2012 NOFAs for Discretionary Programs.* Accessed January 12, 2016. http://portal.hud .gov/hudportal/documents/huddoc?id=2012gensecNOFA.pdf.

U.S. Department of Justice (DOJ). 2009. *The Matthew Shepard and James Byrd, Jr., Hate Crimes Prevention Act of 2009.* Accessed January 12, 2016. http://www.justice.gov/crt/matthew-shepard-and-james-byrd -jr-hate-crimes-prevention-act-2009-0.

U.S. Supreme Court. 2003. Lawrence et al. v. Texas, No. 02-102. Accessed January 13, 2016. http://caselaw.findlaw.com/us-supreme-court/ 539/558.html.

Vermont Ethics Network. 2011a. "Decision-Making Capacity." Accessed January 27, 2016. http://www.vtethicsnetwork.org/decisionmaking .html.

———. 2011b. "Health Care Ethics: Overview and Basics." Accessed January 27, 2016. http://www.vtethicsnetwork.org/ethics.html.

———. 2011c. "Importance of Goals for Care." Accessed January 27, 2016. http://www.vtethicsnetwork.org/importance_of_goals.html.

Victoria Hospice Society. 2001. *Palliative Performance Scale Version 2 (PPSv2)*. Accessed May 28, 2016. http://www.npcrc.org/files/news/palliative_performance_scale_PPSv2.pdf.

Wenzel, H. 2015. *Legal Issues for LGBT Caregivers*. Family Caregiver Alliance, National Center on Caregiving. Accessed March 14, 2016. https://www.caregiver.org/legal-issues-lgbt-caregivers.

WGBH Educational Foundation. 2011. "Timeline: Milestones in the American Gay Rights Movement." Produced in connection with *American Experience* television series. Accessed January 12, 2016. http://www.pbs.org/wgbh/americanexperience/features/timeline/stonewall/.

White, Patrick. 2013. "Use of 'Cisgender' Perpetuates Problematic Dichotomy." *Kansas State Collegian*, April 15, 2013. Accessed April 28, 2016. http://www.kstatecollegian.com/2013/04/15/use-of-cisgender-perpetuates-problematic-dichotomy/.

Williamson, D., J. Lesandrini, and J. Kamdar. 2016. "Incapacitated and Surrogateless Patients: Decision Making for the Surrogateless Patient: An Attempt to Improve Decision Making." *The American Journal of Bioethics* 16 (2): 83–85.

Wittenberg, E., B. Ferrell, J. Goldsmith, T. Smith, M. Glajchen, and G. Handzo, eds. 2015. *Textbook of Palliative Care Communication*. New York: Oxford University Press.

World Health Organization (WHO). 2006. *Defining Sexual Health: Report of a Technical Consultation on Sexual Health, 28–31 January 2002, Geneva*. Geneva: World Health Organization. Accessed March 20, 2016. http://www.who.int/reproductivehealth/publications/sexual_health/defining_sexual_health.pdf.

―――. 2010. *Developing Sexual Health Programmes: A Framework for Action*. Geneva: World Health Organization. Accessed January 11, 2016. http://apps.who.int/iris/bitstream/10665/70501/1/WHO_RHR_HRP_10.22_eng.pdf.

―――. 2016a. "What Do We Mean by 'Sex' and 'Gender'?" Accessed January 11, 2016. http://apps.who.int/gender/whatisgender/en/.

―――. 2016b. "Genomic Resource Centre: Gender and Genetics." Accessed January 7, 2016. http://www.who.int/genomics/gender/en/index1.html.

World Professional Association for Transgender Health. 2012. *Standards of Care for the Health of Transsexual, Transgender, and Gender Nonconforming People*. Accessed January 26, 2016. http://www.wpath.org/uploaded_files/140/files/Standards%20of%20Care,%20V7%20Full%20Book.pdf.

Wynn, S. 2014. "Decisions by Surrogates: An Overview of Surrogate Consent Laws in the United States." *Bifocal: A Journal of the American Bar Association Commission on Law and Aging* 36 (1): 10–14.

Yennurajalingam, S., and E. Bruera, eds. 2016. *Oxford American Handbook of Hospice and Palliative Medicine and Supportive Care*. New York: Oxford University Press.

ABOUT THE CONTENT EXPERT REVIEWERS

Each expert reviewer who consulted on the content of this volume provided a brief biographical statement incorporating the name, pronouns, and honorific of their choice. This practice is intended to model the way in which we should support patients and families as they define and present themselves to the world.

Reverend Vonshelle J. Beneby, MDiv, has been in ministry since 1992, and was ordained in the United Church of Christ in 2009. Vonshelle is a chaplain/psychosocial support coordinator for VITAS Healthcare in Volusia and Flagler Counties, Florida. Vonshelle assesses and provides for the spiritual needs of patients, families, caregivers, and staff through pastoral care, spiritual counseling, and bereavement services. Vonshelle is a member of the VITAS Ethics and Quality Assessment Committees. Vonshelle is a certified trainer and lecturer at VITAS and the recipient of multiple Employee of the Year Awards for Outstanding Chaplain Service. In local churches, Vonshelle is involved with pastoral care, planning and participating in worship services, preaching, and liturgical/interpretive dance. Vonshelle also serves as a consultant and leads discussions and workshops on ways churches may become more inclusive, open, and affirming.

Constance Dahlin, ANP-BC, ACHPN, FPCN, FAAN, is an advanced practice registered nurse with extensive administrative, clinical, and academic experience in hospice and palliative care. Ms. Dahlin is director of professional practice at the Hospice and Palliative Nurses Association (HPNA), a consultant to the Center to Advance Palliative Care for its community-based initiative, a palliative nurse practitioner at North Shore Medical Center in Massachusetts, and co-principal investigator on a project designed to provide primary palliative care education to rural and community APRNs. She serves on the national faculty for the End-of-Life Nursing Education Consortium. She is cochair of the Massachusetts Comprehensive Cancer and Control Network Palliative Care Workgroup and the Circle of Life Committee. She cofounded a pioneering academic palliative care service, where she was clinical director and codirector of the developing outpatient clinic. She was clinical director of an urban hospice and coordinator of a community hospice and home health agency. Ms. Dahlin is a clinical associate professor at the Massachusetts General Hospital Institute of Health Professions and on the faculty of the Harvard Medical School Center for Palliative Care. She is editor of the second and third editions of the National Consensus Project for Quality Palliative Care text *Clinical Practice Guidelines for Quality Palliative Care.* She is coeditor of the recently published *Advanced Practice Palliative Nursing* and the first and second editions of the Hospice and Palliative Nurses Association's *Core Curriculum for the Advanced Hospice and Palliative Registered Nurse.* She served as board president of the Hospice and Palliative Nurses Association and on the National Quality Forum

Hospital Efficiency Task Force, Measure Applications Partnership. Ms. Dahlin is an ally committed to the delivery of high-quality palliative care to LGBTQ people and their families.

Gary Gardia, MEd, MSW, LCSW, began his career as a volunteer more than thirty years ago. He has since worked in many capacities and led a variety of teams and departments. Gary received the Heart of Hospice Award from the National Hospice and Palliative Care Organization (NHPCO) for developing innovative programs to meet the needs of caregivers and the bereaved. Gary has also worked as a psychotherapist in private practice with a specialty in grief and loss, personal growth and development, and substance abuse, as well as in offering guidance for people diagnosed with serious illnesses. For more than seven years Gary served in leadership positions with NHPCO, including as the national section leader for Volunteers and Volunteer Managers and section leader for Social Workers. He recently wrote and taught an eight-month all-online course entitled Post-MSW Palliative Care Certificate and an eight-week course entitled Critical Palliative Care Skills for Social Workers that have been taken by social workers worldwide. Gary is a frequent presenter and keynote speaker at state and national conferences, and provides education, coaching, and retreats for hospital palliative care programs, hospice services, and other businesses.

Judi T. Haberkorn, PhD, MSW, MPH, MBA, is a health care practitioner with more than twenty years of experience in health care and social services. Dr. Haberkorn has served as both an assistant professor and a health care training executive. Dr. Haberkorn has spent nearly ten years in the hospice field and considers it an honor to work with patients in end-of-life care.

Noelle Marie C. Javier, MD, is a trained internist, geriatrician, and hospice and palliative care specialist who also serves as a faculty member at the Icahn School of Medicine at Mount Sinai in New York. She is a longtime advocate and champion for the provision of high-quality and holistic medical care to the marginalized members of society, including older adults, the indigent population, and members of the LGBTQ population. As an empowered minority woman of Asian descent and transgender experience, she also understands firsthand the unique set of care needs affecting this population. She has taken part in and continues to promote culturally sensitive health care education and training in local and regional settings.

Chaplain Sam Mullen ministers in an interfaith capacity in hospice chaplaincy with VITAS Healthcare, where he has been a staff chaplain for four years. After serving fifteen years as an evangelical pastor, Sam came out as gay and is now actively involved in advocacy for the LGBTQ community. Sam has completed two units of clinical pastoral education, is certified as a grief coach, and has worked with several gay hospice patients. Sam also leads bereavement support groups for LGBTQ people in his area.

Martha Rutland, DMin, is director of clinical pastoral education at VITAS Healthcare. She is a certified supervisor with the Association for Clinical Pastoral Education and a certified chaplain with the Association of Professional Chaplains; she holds a doctor of ministry from Chicago Theological Seminary. Martha is also an ordained minister in the United Methodist Church.

ABOUT THE AUTHOR

Kimberly Acquaviva, PhD, MSW, CSE, is a tenured associate professor at the George Washington University School of Nursing. She works as a social worker teaching within a school of nursing, and her scholarship is interdisciplinary and collaborative. Kim's scholarly work focuses on lesbian, gay, bisexual, and transgender aging and end-of-life issues, and her clinical work has been with patients and families facing life-limiting illnesses in both hospital and hospice settings.

Kim has a PhD in human sexuality education from the University of Pennsylvania Graduate School of Education, an MSW from the University of Pennsylvania School of Social Policy and Practice (formerly the School of Social Work), and a BA in sociology from the University of Pennsylvania College of Arts and Sciences. She attained certification as a Certified Sexuality Educator (CSE) through the American Association of Sexuality Educators, Counselors, and Therapists.

Kim lives in Washington, DC, with her wife, Kathy, their teenage son, Greyson, and their three dogs, Dizzy, Zippy, and Mitzi.

www.kimberly-acquaviva.com

INDEX

droppers, 174–175 *t. 8.4*

Drotos, Kunga Nyima, 130–131, 151

durable power of attorney. *See* health care power of attorney (DPOA)

dying/death: attitudes/beliefs about, 6–7; safe/comfortable, questions about, 82–83 *t. 4.2*

Dying in America (IOM), xiv–xv

dysphagia, 165 *t. 8.2*

dyspnea, 165 *t. 8.2*

eating, 160–161 *t. 8.1*

edema, 166 *t. 8.2*

Edgman-Levitan, S., 92

Edmonton Functional Assessment Tool, 75

Edmonton Symptom Assessment System, 75

education. *See* patient/family education

educational materials, 51–52

Eisenhower, Dwight D., 41–42

electric razors, 131

electronic record keeping, 56–58

Elwyn, G., 91, 92

emergency room visits, 167 *t. 8.2*

emotional cutoff, 108

emotional distress, 187–188, 203, 225

emotions: defined, 225; knowing, 3, 11–13, 20

empathic behaviors, 15, 16 *t. 1.1*, 225

empathy, 226

employee benefits/orientation/training, 214–215, 218, 226

employment discrimination, 40–42, 226

employment laws, 212

Employment of Homosexuals and Other Sex Perverts in Government (U.S. Senate report), 40

employment policies, 50–51

end-of-life care, 79–83

end-of-life personal development, 189–192

end-stage disease, 226

end-stage disease progression, education about, xxiii, 159, 164, 165–167 *t. 8.2*, 179

environmental risks, xxiii, 125 *t. 6.2*, 127–132, 133

environmental/safety assessment, xxiii, 226

Epiphaniou, E., 51

Equal Pay Act (1963), 212

Erickson-Schroth, Laura, 24

ethical principles, xxiii, 137–139, 144, 146, 154, 226

ethics, codes of, 207–209, 218

ethnicity: barriers to care and, 39, 40; in institutional nondiscrimination statements, 210–211

euthanasia, 105

Executive Order 10450, 41–42

existential concerns, 200 *t. 9.3*

expected outcomes, 117–118, 118 *t. 6.1*, 132, 133, 226

exsanguination, 175

eye contact, 57, 87, 226

eye-level approach, 226

facilitating behaviors, 15, 16 *t. 1.1*, 226

family: advance care planning and, 141–142; bereavement care, 202; confidentiality and, 152; coping mechanisms, 188–189; emotional distress of, 187–188; end-of-life care questions for, 79–83, 80–83 *t. 4.2*; estranged, 108–109, 144; goals for care, 117, 119–120, 132, 134; institutional inclusiveness and, 210; presence at history/physical exams, 59, 60–62; questions about, 67–68; relationships within, chapter activity for, 112; spiritual/existential distress of, 198–199; types of, 58–59; as unit of care, 115, 132, 141. *See also* patient/family education; shared decision-making process

family dynamics: assumptions about, 109, 111, 188, 203; mapping, 110–111;

shared decision-making process and, 107–110, 111–112

Family and Medical Leave Act, xxii

family meetings: core principles for, 121; discussion questions, 112; Family Perspectives, 60; first, conducting/coordinating, xxi, 58–62, 121; hypothetical scenario, 103–106; setting up, 100–103

family of choice: bereavement care, 202; defined, 58–59, 226–227; discussion questions, 88–89; first family meeting and, 59; questions about, 67, 68; shared decision-making process, 95–97

family of origin: assumptions about, 203; bereavement care, 202; confidentiality and, 152; defined, 58–59, 227; discussion questions, 88–89; first family meeting and, 59; questions about, 67–68; shared decision-making process, 95–97

Family Perspectives: family meetings, 60; hospice care, 61–62

fatigue, 66, 171 t. 8.3, 179, 227

fear, 227

Federal Civil Rights Act (1964), 212

feeding, 178

Fenway Institute, 29, 30

Ferrell, B., xiv–xv, 64, 66, 92

FICA Spiritual History Tool, 65, 70, 197, 227

financial difficulties, 125 t. 6.2

Fins, J. J., 91

Five-Dimension Assessment Model: about (overview), 87–88; activity using, 89; additional questions, 79–83, 80–83 t. 4.2, 85 t. 4.3; Anticipatory Planning for Death (Dimension 5), 77–78; care plan development and, 115–116, 120–121; components of, 66, 87, 227; Decision Making (Dimension 4), 76–77, 183; development of, 64–66; discussion questions, 88–89; Functional Activities/Symptoms (Dimension 3), 73–76, 87, 159, 168, 183; Illness/Treatment Summary (Dimension 2), 71–73; Patient as

Person (Dimensions 1A/1B), 67–71, 79, 195–197; using, 66–67, 87

Florida, 42, 44

focused history, 227

Fromme, E., 59, 109

funeral directive, 148–149

funerals, 78, 150

Gafni, A., 92

Gardia, Gary, 120, 191

gauze, 172, 176 t. 8.5

Gawande, Atul, 137

gay men: with AIDS, 8–9, 119; barriers to care, 39; defined, 31; discrimination against, 40–42; knowledge gaps about, 23; marriages of, 84; Provider Perspectives, 8–9

gender: about (overview), 22–23; defined, 24, 34; questions about, 11, 29–30; sex vs., 24–25, 34

gender-affirmation surgery, 87, 227–228

gender discordance, xxi, 23, 28, 228

gender dysphoria, xxi, 23, 28, 43, 228

Gendered Innovations, 24

gender expression/presentation: about (overview), xxi, 22–23; defined, 25, 228; gender identity vs., 25–26; in institutional nondiscrimination statements, 50–51, 210–213, 218

gender identity: about (overview), xxi, 22–23, 34–35; barriers to care and, 39–40; in comprehensive histories, 62; confidentiality about, 152–154, 155; defined, 25, 34, 228; discussion questions, 35–36; employment discrimination on basis of, 42; gender expression/presentation vs., 25–26; housing discrimination on basis of, 43–44; in institutional nondiscrimination statements, 50–51, 210–213, 218; in intake forms/processes, 215–216; patient treatment according to, 87; physical examinations and, 86–87; questions about, 29–30, 65–66; sexual orientation vs., 28–29, 34 gender identity disorder, 43

gender nonconformity: about (overview), 22–23; barriers to care and, 39–40; defined, 26–28, 228; *DSM* classification status, 43; housing discrimination on basis of, 43–44

gender pronouns: confidentiality and, 155; gender-neutral, xxi, 27; Provider Perspectives, 12; questions about, 11, 67, 216

genderqueer, 228

gender reassignment, 228. *See also* gender-affirmation surgery

gender transition guidelines, 214

genograms, 110, 111–112, 228

GenoPro, 110, 112

Georgia, 42, 44, 45

Geriatric Palliative Care (Chai et al.), xiv–xv

Gibson, S., xv

Gill, J., 92

Gladding, S., 188, 189

Gleason, K. M., 168–172

goals for care, xxi, 117–121, 132–133, 228

Gollance, Richard, 57

Griebling, T., 33

grief/grieving: bereavement care, 202–203; concerns about, 200 *t. 9.3;* defined, 228; expected outcomes, 124 *t. 6.2*, 126 *t. 6.2*, 127 *t. 6.2;* questions about, 82–83 *t. 4.2*

guilt, 200 *t. 9.3*, 228

hair dryers, 131

Harding, R., 51, 202

hate crime laws, 45

hate crimes, 45–47

Hawkins, Jennifer, xxii

Hay, A., xviii

health care: equality in, in institutions, 214; ethical principles and, 137–139; legal issues in decision making, 148–149, 155

health care ethics, 228–229. *See also* ethical principles

health care power of attorney (DPOA): author's experience, 109–110; defined, 143–144, 229; family dynamics and, 111; hypothetical scenario involving, 94, 96–97; importance of, for unmarried LGBTQ people, 144, 154; legal/financial POA vs., 143, 146

health care proxy, 143, 224, 229

health insurance, 50

Health Insurance Portability and Accountability Act (HIPAA), 152, 155, 184; Privacy Rule (45 CFR 164.510B), 68

hearing impairments, 60, 121

hemoptysis, 175

Henrickson, M., 59

heterosexuality: bereavement care, 203; casual self-disclosures of, 17; defined, 31, 229

Hilliard, Russell, 184–186

HIPAA. *See* Health Insurance Portability and Accountability Act (HIPAA)

HIV, 210–211

hobbies, 69

home care, oxygen use in, 129–131, 133, 138

homelessness, 44

homophobia, 40–42

homosexuality, 31, 42–43, 229. *See also* gay men; lesbians

hope, 183, 188–189, 203–204, 229

hopelessness, 200 *t. 9.3*

hormone therapy, 50, 72

Hospice and Palliative Credentialing Center (HPCC), xix

Hospice and Palliative Nurses Association (HPNA), 98–99

hospice care: care plan and, 111; defined, 229; Family Perspectives, 61–62; institutional barriers to, 50–52; LGBTQ outreach and, 209–210; myths/misperceptions about, 48–50, 52; patient goals of care in, 121–122; Patient

intersex, 24–25

isolation, 200 *t. 9.3*

Javier, Noelle Marie C., 119

Johansen, M., 92

Johnson, S., xviii

Joint Commission, 29

justice, 138, 154, 226, 230

Kaleem, J., 199

Kallio, Jay, 41

Kamdar, J., 144

Kansas, 42, 44

Karnofsky Performance Scale, 75

Kentucky, 42, 44

Kerr, M., 107–108

Knight, S., 63, 64, 65, 66, 197

Krayger, Nick, 61–62

Kroenke, K., 75

Kübler-Ross, Elisabeth, 191

labor laws, 212

Lambda Legal, 39, 40, 53, 148–149, 150, 210, 215

lancets, 172, 176 *t. 8.5*

language, inclusive, 195–197, 197 *t. 9.2*, 199–201, 204. *See also* gender pronouns

Laramie (Wyo.), 45

LaRocca-Pitts, M., 192–193

Lau, D. T., 168

laughter, 18

lavender family, 59

"Lavender Scare," 40–42

Lawton, A., 59, 109

legal decisions, 76–77

legal issues, xxiii, 125 *t. 6.2*, 137, 147–152, 155. *See also* power of attorney

Legare, F., 92

Lesandrini, J., 144

lesbians: barriers to care, 39; bereavement care, 202; bisexual women and, 32; defined, 31, 230; discrimination against, 40–42; hypothetical shared decision-making scenario involving, 94–107; knowledge gaps about, 23

leukemia, 175

LGBTQ-inclusive practice: as active choice, xiii–xiv; assessment model developed for, 64, 65–66; in codes of ethics, 207–209; competencies for, xvii–xx; comprehensive history in, 55; conceptual understanding needed for, 23–24; education for, 51–52; historical barriers to care and, 40; Provider Perspectives, xxii; research publications and, xiv–xvi; self-awareness needed for, 3; shifting to, xvi–xvii. *See also* institutional inclusiveness

LGBTQ people: assumptions about, 109, 111, 188; criminalization of, 44; as employees, 214–215; family dynamics of, 108–109, 188; hate crimes against, 45–47; hospice/palliative care concerns of, 49–50; institutional bridges to, 209–217, 218; knowledge gaps about, 23–24; legal issues, 147–152; as "mentally ill," 42–43; in research publications, xiv–xvi; self-disclosures ("coming out") by, 38–39; smoking rate among, 129–131, 133; unmarried, and power of attorney, 144; U.S. discrimination history, 40–47, 52

life completion/closure, developmental tasks associated with, xxiii, 189–192, 230–231

life review, 231

lighters, 131

lip balm, 131

listening, 57, 87, 231

living will, 144–145, 146–147, 231

lotions, oil-based, 131

Louisiana, 42, 44

Lux-Sullivan, Holly, 84

lymphatic obstruction, 166 *t. 8.2*

Lynch, M., 95, 98

Nebraska, 42, 44

neurological examination, 86

Neville, S., 59

nonadherence, 9

noncompliance, 9

nondiscrimination statements, 50–51, 210–214, 215, 218–219

nonmaleficence, 138, 154, 226, 231

nonverbal communication, 231

normalization, 231

North American Nursing Diagnosis Association, 236

North Carolina, 42, 44, 45

North Dakota, 42, 44, 45

nurses: code of ethics of, 208, 218; communication skills of, 15, 57; comprehensive histories compiled by, 57; FICA Spiritual History Tool as used by, 65; at first family meeting, 58; goals for care, 122; hospice/palliative care competencies, xviii, xix; interactions with patients, 4; as interdisciplinary/interprofessional team members, 230; patient/family education by, 159, 164, 172, 179; physical examination by, 85–86; psychosocial/spiritual issues and, 183–184, 187, 189, 194, 196 *t. 9.1*; shared decision-making process and, 93, 94, 95, 97–99, 102, 103, 106–107; symptom management and, 95; team meetings led by, 123. *See also* interdisciplinary/interprofessional teams

nursing, xvii

nutritional supplements, 72

obituaries, 78, 150

Ohio, 42, 44, 45

Oklahoma, 42, 44, 45

open posture, 231–232

organ donation, 150

Orlando (Fla.) mass shooting (2016), 45–47

Otis-Green, S., xiv–xv, 34, 64

"outing," 50

out-of-hospital provider/physician/medical order for life-sustaining treatment (POLST/MOLST), 76, 146, 232

outreach, 51, 52

Oxford Textbook of Palliative Medicine (Cherny et al.), xiv–xv, 64

Oxford Textbook of Palliative Nursing (Ferrell, Coyle, and Paice), xiv–xv, 64, 66

Oxford Textbook of Palliative Social Work (Altilio and Otis-Green), xiv–xv, 64

oxygen, home use of, 129–131, 133, 138

Paice, J., xiv–xv, 64, 66

pain: assessment instruments, 75; defined, 232; during end-stage disease progression, 166 *t. 8.2*

pain management, xxiii, 159, 168, 169–171 *t. 8.3*, 179, 232

palliative care: care plan and, 111; defined, 232; institutional barriers to, 50–52; LGBTQ outreach and, 209–210; myths/misperceptions about, 48, 49–50, 52; patient goals of care in, 121–122; shared decision making in, 91, 101 *t. 5.1, t. 5.2*, 111

Palliative Care Fast Facts (Palliative Care Network of Wisconsin), 75

Palliative Care Network of Wisconsin, 75

palliative care professionals: advance care planning and, 141–142; FICA Spiritual History Tool and, 65; research publications for, xiv–xvi

Palliative Performance Scale Version 2, 75

palliative sedation: decision-making guidelines, 102; defined, 95, 232; ethics of, 97–99; misconceptions about, 105; risks/benefits of, 99–100; shared decision making regarding, 91, 94

"Palliative Sedation Position Statement" (AAHPM), 98

pansexuality, 232

patient: ADLs, 62; advance care planning and, 141–142; advance directives, 62; -centered terminology, 10; coping mechanisms, 188–189; emotional distress of, 187–188; end-of-life care questions for, 79–83, 80–83 t. 4.2; goals for care, 58, 62, 117–121, 132–133, 134; knowing, 3, 10–11, 20; as person, xxi, 55, 64, 65–66, 67–71; power imbalances with, 9–10, 19–20; quality of life, 62; right to self-determination of, 9; sexual health assessments of, 33–34; spiritual/existential distress of, 198–200; as unit of care, 115, 132, 141. *See also* patient/family education

Patient and Family Outcomes-Focused Inquiry for Developing Goals for Care, 79–83, 80–83 t. 4.2, 122, 233

Patient and Family Outcomes-Focused Inquiry for Interdisciplinary Teams, xxi–xxiii, 83, 122–123, 124–127 t. 6.2, 133, 233

patient-care skills, assessing/teaching, xxiii, 159–164, 160–163 t. 8.1, 178–179, 233

patient-centered approach, 233

patient/family education: about (overview), xxiii, 158–159, 178–179; activity involving, 180; discussion questions, 179–180; end-stage disease progression, xxiii, 164, 165–167 t. 8.2, 179; imminent death signs/symptoms, xxiii, 159, 172, 175, 177–178 t. 8.6, 178; importance of, 178; medical supply disposal, xxiii, 172, 176 t. 8.5, 179; medication management, xxiii, 168–172, 173–175 t. 8.4, 179; pain/symptom management, xxiii, 168, 169–171 t. 8.3, 179; patient-care skills, xxiii, 159–164, 160–163 t. 8.1, 178–179

Patient Health Questionnaire PHQ-9, 75

Patient Perspectives: bisexuality, 32; homophobia, 41; hospice care, 49

Patient Self-Determination Act (1990), 234

Paul, R., 5

Paxton, S., 48

PEACE Project, 75–76

Pediatric Palliative Care (Ferrell), xiv–xv

Peek, M., 92

Pennsylvania, 42, 44, 45

pericardial effusion, 167 t. 8.2

petroleum jelly, 131

PFLAG, 188

pharmacy benefits, 48

physical examination: defined, 233; family presence at, 59, 60–62; as first meeting focus, 58; of palliative care/hospice patients, 85–86; of transgender patients, 86–87

physicians: code of ethics of, 208–209, 218; communication skills of, 15, 57; comprehensive histories compiled by, 57; FICA Spiritual History Tool as used by, 65; at first family meeting, 58; goals for care, 122; hospice/palliative care competencies, xvii–xix; interactions with patients, 4; as interdisciplinary/interprofessional team members, 230; legal issues, 76, 229; patient/family education by, 159, 164, 172, 179; physical examination by, 85–86; primary-care, 48, 99, 100, 106, 152, 169–171 t. 8.3; psychosocial/spiritual issues and, 183–184, 187, 189, 194, 196 t. 9.1; shared decision-making process and, 92, 93, 94, 98–99, 102, 103, 104–107; team meetings led by, 123. *See also* interdisciplinary/interprofessional teams

pills, 175 t. 8.4

pleural effusion, 167 t. 8.2

pneumonia, 165 t. 8.2

Portenoy, R., 75

"Position Statement: Palliative Sedation at the End of Life" (HPNA), 98

postural hypotension, 166 t. 8.2

power imbalances, 9–10, 19–20, 233

power of attorney, 143, 146. *See also* health care power of attorney (DPOA)

prejudgments, knowing, 4–5

presence, 233

pressure ulcers, 167 t. 8.2

primary care providers, 48, 99, 100, 106, 152, 169–171 t. 8.3

Principles of Analgesic Use in the Treatment of Acute Pain and Cancer Pain (American Pain Society), 75

Principles of Biomedical Ethics (Beauchamp and Childress), 137–138

prognosis, 62, 76, 233

property ownership, 149–152, 155

Provider Perspectives: advance care planning, 140; barriers to care, 51; care plan, 119, 120, 130–131; comprehensive histories, 57; gender pronouns, 12; home hospice care, 84; legal issues, 151; LGBTQ-inclusive practice, xxii; patients with AIDS, 8–9; psychosocial/spiritual issues, 191, 198, 201; safety risks, 130–131

psychological distress, 187–188, 234

psychosocial assessment, xxiii, 183–186, 203, 234

psychosocial history, 62, 94, 234

psychosocial/spiritual issues: about (overview), xxiii, 182–183, 203–204; activity involving, 205; bereavement care, 202–203, 204; despair/hope/meaning, 188–189, 203–204; discussion questions, 204–205; emotional distress, 187–188, 203; in inpatient setting, 195, 196 *fig. 9.1;* language for, 195–197, 197 *t. 9.2,* 199–201, 204; life completion/closure, xxiii, 189–192; Provider Perspectives, 191, 198, 201; psychosocial assessment, 183–186, 203; spiritual concerns, 200 *t. 9.3;* spiritual/existential assessment, 192–195, 203, 204; spiritual/existential distress, 197–200, 204

Puchalski, Christina, 65, 69, 194–195, 196 *fig. 9.1,* 199, 200 *t. 9.3*

Pulse nightclub mass shooting (Orlando, Fla.; 2016), 45–47

quality of life, 62, 234

questions, relevant vs. intrusive, 83, 85 *t. 4.3*

Quintana, Vicki, 12

race: barriers to care and, 39, 40; in institutional nondiscrimination statements, 210–211

rainbow "ally" pins, 16–17

rapport, 234

Rawlings, D., 59

reactions, knowing/controlling, 3, 13–14, 20

reconciliation, 200 *t. 9.3*

reflection, 234

registered nurses (RNs): code of ethics of, 208, 218; communication skills of, 15, 57; comprehensive histories compiled by, 57; FICA Spiritual History Tool as used by, 65; at first family meeting, 58; goals for care, 122; hospice/palliative care competencies, xviii, xix; interactions with patients, 4; as interdisciplinary/interprofessional team members, 230; patient/family education by, 159, 164, 172, 179; physical examination by, 85–86; psychosocial/spiritual issues and, 183–184, 187, 189, 194, 196 *t. 9.1;* shared decision-making process and, 93, 94, 95, 97–99, 102, 103, 106–107; symptom management and, 95; team meetings led by, 123. *See also* interdisciplinary/interprofessional teams

Rehabilitation Act (1973), 212

relaxation techniques, 179

religious beliefs: concerns about, 200 *t. 9.3;* family dynamics and, 96–97, 103–104; funeral planning and, 150; in institutional nondiscrimination statements, 210–211; LGBTQ-inclusive practice and, xiii; patient negative experiences with, 88; Provider Perspectives, xxii; questions about, 69, 70; spiritual/existential distress and, 198–200; spiritual/existential history and, 88. *See also* spiritual/existential *entries*

research publications, xiv–xvi

resource deficits, 125 *t. 6.2*

restroom policies, 214

risk-benefit discussion tool for shared decision making, 101 *t. 5.1, t. 5.2*

risk management, 7

rituals, 78

Ross, D., 94

safety risks, xxiii, 125 *t. 6.2,* 127–133

same-sex marriage, 84, 151